"[An] uncommon, contemplative novel . . . eloquent, evocative writing."
—*The Orlando Sentinel*

"Entrancing . . . beguiling . . . Brown's dramatic and multifaceted tale doesn't simply rest on the intrigue of a moment in American medical history when premature infants were displayed as 'freaks.' While she navigates readers through the complex intersections of medicine, social responsibility and free enterprise, her lyrical, touching story succeeds on the strength of her affection for the characters she accords dignity and a yearning for love."
—*Publishers Weekly*

"Another unexpected little jewel from Brown...This is a moving story about complex, interesting characters who love deeply, and it is wonderful. Most highly recommended."
—*Library Journal* (starred review)

"She vividly re-creates the 'vast, perplexing, hallucinatory landscape' of the fair . . . well-researched."
—*The New York Times Book Review*

"A bittersweet, compassionate story . . . Her rich characterizations and descriptions bring readers back in time while the truly rendered emotions are universal." —*The Dallas Morning News*

"Brown tells her story with great delicacy, giving an otherworldly, luminous air to a tawdry setting and great dignity to her characters."
—*Kirkus Reviews*

"A meditation on why we live and who we love and what we hope for . . . Brown conveys wonderfully the size, scope and noise of the fair. . . . Her details are remarkable."—*Milwaukee Journal Sentinel*

"Carrie Brown is a writer of uncommon gifts: lovely, lyrical language and startling originality."
—Lee Smith

continued . . .

"Beguiling."   —*St. Louis Post-Dispatch*

"Her writing, called lyrical so often it sounds like a cliché, has the misty quality of a dream, with unknown events at the hazy edges, characters who are very real and yet removed by a time-frosted looking glass. Brown uses ordinary words in an extraordinary way. The people are remarkable and their situations often transcendent, but it is the way she tells it that is distinctive. The telling *is* lyrical—so much so that you can hear the music in the background. . . . With a delicate, masterful hand, Brown has created a thing of beauty and wonder."   —*Salisbury (NC) Post*

"Suffused with a warm and sympathetic intelligence—yet one that never slops over into sentimentality. Her characters are vivid, believable and engaging, but never maudlin."   —*Chicago Tribune*

"Fans of Caleb Carr will see in this story by Carrie Brown a similar talent for creating a historic scene that has more than its share of the bizarre."   —*Amarillo (TX) Sunday News-Globe*

"Once you start this book you find yourself absolutely fascinated with the world it presents. . . . I heartily recommend it for some unusual and fascinating reading."   —*The Pinehurst (NC) Pilot*

"A luminous, exceptional book."   —*Greensboro News & Record*

"Brown's sensuous voice lets the reader feel the heat of a Chicago summer and know the fear of the young father lost in the confusion and crowds of the world's fair. . . . A fascinating and meaningful look into the world of alternate family systems and the power of love."   —*Boston Herald*

Also by Carrie Brown

Rose's Garden
Lamb in Love

The
Hatbox Baby

◼

A NOVEL BY

Carrie Brown

𝕭

BERKLEY BOOKS, NEW YORK

ℬ

A Berkley Book
Published by The Berkley Publishing Group
A division of Penguin Putnam Inc.
375 Hudson Street
New York, New York 10014

PRINTING HISTORY
Algonquin Books of Chapel Hill hardcover edition / September 2000
Berkley trade paperback edition / June 2002

Visit our website at
www.penguinputnam.com

Library of Congress Cataloging-in-Publication Data

Brown, Carrie, 1959–
The hatbox baby / Carrie Brown.
p. cm.
ISBN 0-425-18465-X
1. Century of Progress International Exposition (1933–1934 : Chicago, Ill.)—
Fiction. 2. Physician and patient—Fiction. 3. Infants (Premature)—
Fiction. 4. Chicago (Ill.)—Fiction. 5. Pediatricians—Fiction.
6. Neonatology—Fiction. I. Title.

PS3552.R68529 H3 2002
813'.54—dc21   2001052930

PRINTED IN THE UNITED STATES OF AMERICA

10 9 8 7 6 5 4 3 2 1

For John

And for the children,

Olivia, Molly, and Walker,

late, early, and on time

Some are transformed just once

And live their whole lives after in that shape.

—*"Erysichthon," from Tales from Ovid,*

translated by Ted Hughes

CONTENTS

The Hatbox Baby

Carrie Brown

Chicago
The Century of Progress Exposition
June 1933

ONE

The young man with the hatbox under his arm was among the first to arrive at the fair that morning. He stood alone at the top of the Avenue of Flags, under the weak light of the early sun, wondering which way to go. Then, from inside the hatbox held close against his chest, he felt a small, muffled concussion—the baby's foot striking the side of the box. Or the baby's hand? Or head? Or tiny shoulder like a wren's wing, as the child flipped and turned and struggled against the round walls? The movement resounded against his chest, and he felt himself awakening at last from the long night behind him.

It was the first time he'd felt the baby move since Mrs. Hermann had stood up from between his wife's bloody knees and closed the lid over the box and handed it to him. "Take it to that doctor, that one at the fair," she had said. "He's the only one can save it."

He stared straight ahead into the light of the morning—he didn't dare look down—and moved his hand to touch the side of the box. It was like running his palm over Sylvie's swollen belly, the same smooth, round dryness. The same baby inside.

Before him, the empty concourse opened up, a broad runway demarcated on either side by two long lines of flagpoles surmounted by brightly colored pennants. In the insistent wind off Lake Michigan, the flags held taut against a pale sky streaked with declining brush strokes of clouds.

When this was all over, when he had found the doctor and left the baby and come back home again, he would tell Sylvie and Mrs. Hermann about this.

I felt like the last man on earth, he would tell them.

Yet, alone as he felt, the fair was slowly coming to life around him. Solitary preparations were being made behind closed doors and in hidden places. Awake and present, for instance, though invisible to the young man, was a gathering of Hopi Indians, young men and women drinking green tea together in the long, flat shade of a mud hut while repairing the intricate beadwork on their costumes for the butterfly dance to be performed later that day at one-hour intervals.

Also at work at this early hour were the lion tamers, unloading backbreaking hunks of beef and ice from an early delivery truck.

Two waitresses at the Costa Rica Coffee Shop were sleepily measuring and grinding mountains of fragrant beans for the first of the day's many cups of coffee. The driver of a noisy, tenton Pabst Blue Ribbon truck backed slowly down an alley in the Streets of Paris. The aging pianist who played the morning shift at the Baldwin Piano Company's display practiced in the company's suffocating, velvet-draped booth in the empty General Exhibits Pavilion. Under the rising sun, the fire walkers from Darkest Africa silently spread their coals, and at the Maya Temple, the Nunnery of Uxmal, a tiny, barefoot woman in a black dress stepped from the cavelike opening of the temple's entrance and set to sweeping the first of the temple's one hundred steps.

The young man had read about the fair's marvels in the advertisements and the newspaper stories. And everybody in Chicago talked about it. Now here it was, on either side of him, up and down the broad concourses, all the wonders of the world spread out before his eyes — the secrets of science and aeronautics and architecture, the methods of magic and medicine and art and love.

He had read, for instance, about the grim, mechanical pterodactyl groaning from sixteen steel cables in the icy, marble Hall of Science, the creature's shadow falling like a huge webbed foot over farmers from Kansas or Missouri.

And he'd been told about the scientific display from the Baltimore College of Dental Surgery — there they were, George Washington's wooden teeth! Someone had thought to mount them, for purposes of public edification, on a steel pedestal under a glass dome. Alongside were images of George W. before (with original teeth) and George W. after; the improvement certainly was striking, people said.

There were (reportedly) other sights, some troubling. The Deutsches Hygiene Museum's Transparent Man, for instance. In an otherwise empty circular hall, dimly lit and trimmed with a mosaic frieze of inscrutable hieroglyphs, the ten-foot Transparent Man rotated slowly, its arms uplifted in a pose of worship. Its organs — brain, stomach, heart, spleen, liver, gall bladder — were illuminated one by one, a human switchboard.

And there were miracles, too: the fragile Japanese house of polished cedar and bamboo, erected roof-first to the astonishment of all onlookers.

The replica of Mount Vernon fashioned entirely from pearls.

Chains of elephants solemnly moving trees.

Whistler's Mother.

The Nocturnal Gardens of Enchantment.

The seven-foot nine-inch boy from Pennsylvania, fifteen years old and still growing.

Willy Vocalite, the electric robot.

A real, live Ethiopian princess, smoking a cigarette and flicking ash at the feet of the men who came to stare at her.

These were strange sights, to be sure, strange and wondrous, but none was so tempting—his friends said—as the plump, outstretched, freckled arms of the taxi dancers, encouraging passersby onto the floor for a turn or two for a dime. Or the famous fan dancer herself, Caroline Day, her magnificent body glazed with a pink court plaster and dusted with white powder, her breasts a high shelf, rippling like a mirage. She appeared onstage three times a day in a smoky ring of light, her charms winking and vanishing behind a pair of ostrich-feather fans that slowly grazed the blue and indefinite air of the Lido theater.

So much, so many things, all competing for a young man's time and attention, his money, his heart, and his imagination.

And yet this young man had none of those to spare. All he had was a hatbox, and in it his infant son, born too soon.

He walked alone down the thousand yards of the Avenue of Flags, the hatbox held close in his arms, the pennants of geranium red and snow white and sky blue snapping overhead. He had not once looked inside the box since leaving home. He could not bear to see it if it was dead.

He knew that the fair doctor kept his special, tiny babies on display in shiny boxes called incubators. In those incubators, it was said, people could see how nature takes its course deep within the body, how a man can contrive to make a woman's womb. Now his own child had come, nearly three months early, and so he'd traveled obediently—the way a child takes a nickel and goes to buy a loaf of bread for his mother—to find this famous incubator doctor, as his neighbor Mrs. Hermann had proposed. He'd done what he was told to do.

But to him it only felt like his heart was tied up so tightly inside that it hurt, tied up like something bound and gagged for fear it would give itself away. Within minutes of beginning his trip, he had convinced himself that the infant had already died in the hatbox. Mrs. Hermann had said she thought it might; she'd wanted him to be ready if it came to that. But she had succeeded chiefly in making him even more terrified of the child. Wouldn't it move again? He ran his fingers over the box's round side, over the eyelets through which the thin string ran and which admitted air into the hatbox.

"It's enough," Mrs. Hermann had said. "It can breathe, if it will."

Baby?

But he would not open the lid now, not even to peek.

The giant, elongated shadows of early morning fell around him. Passing through zebra stripes of light and dark, he saw fountains and monuments, tents and bivouacs, brightly colored facades and cool, dark passageways. Pausing at the intersection of two wide thoroughfares, he hesitated. A vague instinct prompted him to look up. There in the pale blue sky, between the towering canyon walls of the exposition's architectural monuments, a dirigible balanced lightly on a rack of cloud.

Oh! It was a fantastic thing, such as might be found in a book! An airplane drew a foamy zigzag in the empty air, a child's thick alphabet sloping toward the horizon.

He hoisted the hatbox higher in his arms.

Was it alive or dead? Alive or dead? He did not want to be touching it if it was dead.

Within minutes of his arrival at the fair, the roadways became crowded. People now filled the avenues in groups of two and three and more, their voices high and incoherent-sounding. The fair's bold new buildings, their soaring height and immutable bulk; its barkers and gawkers; its peddlers and converts; its acolytes and innocents—they began to close in around the young man. He stopped, confused.

Which way should he go? Where was the baby doctor?

He walked quickly—*Just go in any direction; it doesn't matter, just keep going*—and soon was soaked. His hair darkened at his temples, and the back of his shirt became stained with sweat. He hurried now past colorful flower gardens, past the reproduction of Abraham Lincoln's rough cabin, past the Belgian glassblowers and the sloe-eyed Moroccans with their piles of brass and leather. He was a fast walker, accustomed since childhood to running if pursued. He would not ask directions; it didn't look smart to be lost.

Though it was still early in the day, he was as hot as if he were running a fever. He wanted a drink of water. At every corner, he saw refreshment for sale—Prohibition was over, beer was back—but it seemed a man could not find just a glass of water, something for nothing. Yet that was what he longed for.

He had eaten nothing before leaving home. He couldn't remember when he had last eaten. The past twenty-four hours blurred behind him, appalling and terrible. He knew what bad luck was (he'd had it all his life, hadn't he?) but he had not been prepared for something so terrible as this, this baby born too soon, this child who now depended on him for its life, to find—quickly, quickly—in this vast, perplexing, hallucinatory landscape, the one man who could save its life.

If there was even a life anymore to be saved.

He tried to walk faster, though it was awkward with the hatbox. He lifted a hand to wipe his forehead. Offshore, Lake Michigan's navy waters shrank and grasped, swallowing the cries of the fair's barkers and the roaring of airplanes, the whip-cracking of pennants high in the sky, the swinging chords of dance music, and the lewd catcalls of men whose wonder had been awakened by the pink, prepossessing breasts of the dancers at the Nudist Colony. The lake's deep waters muffled the sound of crying children, ringing glassware, rolling coins striking a marble tabletop. A leopard's low growl, the chink-chink of silverware, the buzzing, hissing, knitting murmur of conversations in French and Dutch, Javanese and Malay, Swahili and Italian, the broad accents of the Midwest and the expostulations of New Yorkers—all this made a sound as steady and mesmerizing as the five-inch waves of Lake Michigan touching the shore over and over again.

He looked at everything, his eyes darting up and down and to the side, but he kept his ear out for mention of Caroline Day, the fan dancer, because she was the next exhibit over to the baby doctor and was very well known. Famous, in fact. His wife's sister had heard Caroline Day say once that babies wore fewer clothes than she did, and so what was all the fuss?

He wiped his forehead again. A wave of panic traveled up his spine, and a fresh rivulet of sweat ran down and collected at his waist, under his belt. He shifted the hatbox carefully from one arm to the other, careful to keep his eyes from it, as if the thing he held were of no consequence at all, not even worthy of a glance. *What if someone asks what I've got? What if someone stops me?* he thought. *I'll be blamed for it.*

How could it be so hot so early in the morning? He pulled at his collar, wrenching his jaw aside in a grimace that exaggerated, for a second, the ruin of his face. He had an unfortunate collapsed chin, and his hair had darkened since childhood from palest blond to the dull red of natural clay deposits. He had lovely, musical fingers, however—surprisingly long and slender—and the gift of perfect pitch, though he had no way of knowing this. He only knew that he could reach a high note effortlessly and that he liked the sound of his own voice in song. He was happy when he sang.

But his ruined chin—due to a botched tooth extraction two years before—and his slender, cringing air, gave him an untrustworthy appearance, the look of someone who knows he will be presumed guilty. He had minded that his looks had been ruined by the infection in his jaw, but it did not surprise him very much that it had happened. When his wife—short, plump, hopelessly sentimental Sylvie—said she didn't care a whit, when she tossed her head and called him petty, he wondered anew at his good fortune.

Yet, might she mind? One day? Sylvie with her pretty shoes with the pearl buttons, Sylvie with her giggling taste for beer and peanuts, Sylvie with the cheeks that burned red if he kissed her too hard and brushed his rough cheek against hers. She told him he cried too easily "for a man." But he was a hard worker, wasn't he? He'd have done anything for her.

A bouquet of helium balloons leaped from a vendor's hand nearby, startling him. Pink and white and emerald green, they twisted elegantly and freed themselves into the sky.

He was lost.

He had come up into the fairgrounds early that morning by the colossal Field Museum, its gray, imperial edifice set above a broad flight of shallow steps. Though it was only eight in the morning, the crowds moved sluggishly under the climbing sun. He tried, because of the hatbox, to keep his distance from the other passersby: the red-necked, bristle-haired farmers in shiny trousers and soaked shirts; men with their jackets folded over their arms and rings of sweat at their collars; a tall, solemn stranger in fringed buckskin, wiping his face with a cherry-colored rag.

The baby had not moved again; he kept stroking the round side of the box, half hoping to feel a corresponding tap, half afraid to. He tried to dodge carefully through the crowds so as not to jostle the child, but there were so many people, and their movements were so unpredictable. They stopped and started, shuffling along. At one point he found himself stalled in the midst of the International Shoe Buyers Review. The group of white-shirted men with their hand-lettered name tags thronged before the turnstile at the Oriental Village, where a brightly painted and alluring advertisement called all comers to the Slave Mart, an exotic dancing show. Shoulder to shoulder with the shoe buyers, the young man began to feel as if he could not get enough air into his lungs.

His frozen expression and white fingers frightened the fellow nearest to him, an unhappy-looking bachelor from Omaha with a large goiter at his neck. This man glanced over at the thin boy beside him—the boy's eyes straining at their sockets— and then down at the hatbox. A little alarm went off in this man's head at the boy's constricted expression, his hands white-knuckled around the box. What was in that hatbox? Why was the boy holding it that way? Surely, the Omaha bachelor thought nervously, it must contain something bad—something evil, something dangerous—a weapon, or an explosive . . . perhaps a snake! The day before, he had been to see Snakeoid, the man who swallowed live snakes and allowed himself to be bitten by rattlers. Now he was ready to go home.

But before the Omaha bachelor could move himself away from the dangerous-looking young man, the young man himself wrenched free of the crowd of shoe buyers, stumbled into the avenue. He needed water. He needed to find the doctor. His palms had grown slick around the hatbox; his own sweat was staining the cardboard.

He cast about him—ahead was the glorious red-and-gold sunburst of the Bendix Lama Temple of Jehol, twenty-eight thousand meticulously reassembled pieces of an eighteenth-century summer home for Manchu emperors, set down in Chicago on the shore of Lake Michigan.

"My! Isn't it a . . . pretty thing!" said a nearby woman to her companion, fluttering a printed paper fan at her neck.

They looked like sisters, two middle-aged women in brown shoes, sharing an umbrella against the sun. They looked kindly. He was sure they had given their children a whole dollar to spend—sent them off to work the Mechanical Man or push the button that sent hundreds of steel balls falling through pins in the formation of a natural frequency curve. Or perhaps the children would play at African Dips, tossing a ball at a target and dropping a colored man imprisoned in a little cage into a tank of water.

He licked his lips, tore his eyes away from the temple, moved on.

He passed the Odditorium, featuring Siamese twins Mary and Margaret Gibbs, and Johnny Eck, the living half-boy. Nils Nelson, the man with rubber skin, was imprinted over his whole body with a violet imbroglio of lines and etchings, a map to a lost civilization. Armless wonder Martha Morris, standing on an upturned bucket outside a doorway, a small crowd around her, balanced a ball on her nose, flipped it first to her brow and then to the crown of her head.

He skirted the dusty encampment for the Indians—"Two hundred In-juns," a barker cried, "from six different tribes!" Their territory was marked off by totem poles, each with a succession of menacing faces, one atop the other, all staring at him, half-man, bird, or beast.

He passed Midget Village, a nine-hundred-square-foot Bavarian town occupied by eighty-five midgets. One of these stunted men could flip from his hands to his feet, back and forth, back and forth, with the regularity of a metronome. The midget landed suddenly before him, hands planted on his thighs. Tiny geysers of sparkling dust sprang from his soft-soled shoes.

"Watch it," the young man cried, rearing back, clutching the hatbox to his chest.

But the midget had not heard him; his eyes rolled unseeing, the world spinning. He was gone between two tents in a moment.

The young man was breathing hard now; he imagined he felt against his fingertips the last breaths of the child inside the hatbox. He looked up. How miraculous if the doctor should just appear now before him, bending down kindly and extending a hand. But there was no understanding face there. Only a sign: LIFE! the advertisement on the side of the building read. ONE HUNDRED AND EIGHTY REAL EMBRYOS—RAT, SHEEP, OSTRICH—IN PROGRESSIVE STAGES OF DEVELOPMENT.

He stepped back in horror, for he had noticed, in the long, slow, resounding minutes after his son was born, that the baby's tiny ears were limp, without proper definition, as if someone had stepped on the child's temple with a heavy boot. A light covering of fine hair grew over the baby's dusky red body, especially across his shoulders. He could hold it in one hand. It did not look entirely human.

Are we all like this inside our mothers? he had wondered, reeling. *Is this what we look like?*

Also, he noticed: no balls in the little boy's pocket.

He's no good, he'd decided then, turning away from the bloody bed, putting his hands to his temples. *Sylvie's baby is no good. My baby.*

Mrs. Hermann had wrapped the infant herself in a gown that, though intended for a newborn, was comically, pathetically large on this poor weakling of a child.

It was the only thing to be done, they'd agreed, whispering together in the dark kitchen, while Sylvie lay in the bedroom, her face turned to the wall, to the pale patina of dawn collecting like a sand dune up the yellow wall. She would not look at the child. There wasn't any use in seeing it.

"What shall we do?" he'd asked, wringing his hands. "It don't look right. It isn't right, is it? It's too tiny, too tiny. Tell me."

Mrs. Hermann shook her head, not looking at him but cupping the baby's head in her hand, slipping the gown under its spine, small as a fish bone.

Born late in the sixth month of Sylvie's pregnancy, the child was too small and weak to suckle at the breast or even cry. It lay flat, its arms and legs spread out loosely like a small, thin chicken ready for the oven, no more than—what, two or three pounds? But it breathed, surprising Mrs. Hermann, too, he saw. She held it on her lap; he saw with horror that one of her hands encompassed the entirety of it. She sat by, patiently trying to drip sugar water into the infant's mouth from her finger, while he rolled up his soiled shirt and put on a fresh one. He was grateful to her, for she had come right away when he had run downstairs to her door, banged frantically on it.

"It's coming," he'd said when she cracked the door.

She stared at him. "But it's too early," she'd said. "It's—"

"It's coming, I tell you!"

She had looked at him one more moment and then closed her door behind her and run up the stairs ahead of him, her skirts in her fist. He was grateful to her. She knew what to do.

Mrs. Hermann had touched his shoulder when he'd left that morning, but Sylvie would not even open her eyes or let him kiss her good-bye. He'd waited a moment at the bedroom door, hurt and puzzled. Looking vaguely around the room, he was surprised that there wasn't even a picture on the wall. *If we left here tomorrow, there'd be no trace of us,* he thought, and the notion filled him with a cold fear, as if he had failed at some essential test.

When Mrs. Hermann touched him, he had turned to her.

"He's the only one can do anything with it," she repeated, handing him the hatbox and dropping her head on her bosom in prayer. "If God wants it to be."

Everybody in Chicago knew about the baby doctor. Maybe everybody in the country, the world, knew about him. Sylvie's sister Evie had come back from the fair and said she knew it was a thing she would remember her whole life.

"They have tiny little heads—like country apples," she'd said. "*Dear* little things. *Sweet* little things. Oh, Sylvie." And she had leaned over to kiss her sister's swollen belly, looking up into her face. "I hope your baby will be perfect."

Sylvie had managed only a pale smile. She was hot and uncomfortable. Her waist itched; the band of her underwear was too tight.

From the newspaper, Evie had read aloud to them. She had shaken out the page: "'And who would not be stirred by these tiniest of mortals, deaf and feeble and blind, their minute hearts pumping valiantly within their fragile chests? Who does not, looking at them within their glass wombs, consider his own heart and muscle and pronounce it a miracle that he came from such humble beginnings!'

"That's just it," Evie had said, setting down the paper, her eyes bright. And yet her gaze had fallen away from them, onto a distant place. "Those babies, and the one fat woman they call Jolly Irene, all seven hundred pounds of her—like a great big sand castle! Think of the two of them, practically next-door neighbors." She had turned slowly and stared at her sister and brother-in-law. "Aren't we strange!"

Strange, yes. He nodded his head as if Evie were right beside him, talking to him now, keeping him company. So strange.

The soles of his feet seemed to burn through to his bones as he walked. The fair's steaming pavements seemed endless. How long had he been looking now? How many hours walking? Was it near eleven? The baby had been born at 6:43 A.M. He'd looked at his watch, a gift from Sylvie.

He rubbed his hand over his forehead. Sweat stung the tired corners of his eyes—when had he last slept? Not at all last night, when he had sat by Sylvie and tried to hold her hand. He had wanted to run and find a doctor, but she wouldn't let him go, though neither would she let him help her.

"Don't touch me!" she had screamed as he hovered over her.

She had cried, "No, don't look! Don't look!" when he tried to put his hand on her belly and pull the sheet away. "What is happening? It hurts me so much!"

At last, uncharacteristically forceful out of sheer terror, he had let go the corner of the sheet he'd been twisting in his hands and stood up abruptly. "I'm going to get Mrs. Hermann," he'd said, and for once she hadn't argued with him.

Now, standing in the middle of the street, what he wanted, more than anything else, was just a drink of water.

After I give the baby to the doctor, he thought, calmer now, as if there were nothing left to be done or as if the child had already lived and died and passed from their lives like a breeze, *I may see many wonders of the world.*

Couldn't he just put the box down now? Walk away? The notion was sly, a snake.

A jolt went through him; where did such thoughts come from? How were they let in? He gripped the hatbox close as if he could reassure the little baby inside, promise his devotion. Later he would be able to say that he had done the right thing, taking the child to someone who would know what to do with it, the one person for whom this was a specialty, in fact. How lucky they were, really, he told himself, rattling on inside his head. How lucky to be living in Chicago this year, this month, this summer, when this . . . befell them. The great doctor was here, within reach.

But although he believed that the proper way to handle misfortune was to submit to it, to go on and get it over with, in some secret part of his mind now he would be happy to give up this baby—if he could give it up. The child's exquisite frailty, its half-baked look, had terrified him. He wouldn't admit as much to Sylvie; he wouldn't hurt her by showing her how little he wanted this sickly infant. His relief at giving up the baby would have to be his secret. But he *did* want to give it over now, to get rid of it, if it was still alive. He looked down at the box in his hands.

We ought not to be seeing this, he'd thought as Mrs. Hermann knelt between his wife's legs and pulled the tiny creature out.

Poor, poor freakish thing. Suddenly he was braver than he'd been all day. *Doesn't even look like a real baby.*

• • •

The sun struck the zenith overhead, a white-hot token strung up out of reach in the dazzling blue sky. He stepped toward the restaurant. Water splashed from carafes; he saw a child's tongue lick the clear drops of sweat from a glass; he watched a man's throat work up and down like a snake as he threw back his head and drank.

And just at that moment, a friendly voice in his ear, close as a mosquito, said, "Come to see *La Caroline?* Follow me, my friend."

He jerked away from the contagious little whisper, took in a short, wiry man with bulging biceps and a head the shape and weight of a muskmelon, dawdling at his shoulder.

"Now, *everybody* wants to see Caro Day," the little man said cheerfully, beaming up at him. " 'Aw, put a little something over *Sun*day,' they told her. 'You ain't decent company!' " He neatly shifted an unlit cigar to the other corner of his mouth, leaned close. "But I'll swear to you, friend, one hundred dollars to you, *friend*—and I don't care *who* you are—if this little lady has a *shred* over Sunday when she steps up onstage." He opened his hands wide, palms out, as if to say, *See? No tricks.* But a white mouse emerged from his cuff and slid down his wrist, its pink nose twitching. The man clamped his free hand over it, plucked it up by its tail, and returned it serenely to the breast pocket of his shirt. He grinned up at the young man, then ducked coyly out of range. "C'mon, pal. I know a shortcut. Take you to the next show"—he checked a huge pocket watch whisked from his vest. "Starts in two minutes. For a nickel."

The young man with the hatbox stared at this strange apparition, the too-big head and the filthy cravat at the man's neck, his shoes torn open at one toe and flapping. The little man waited, jogging up and down in place with exaggerated effort, running an imaginary race. Then he stopped suddenly and reached over his shoulder as if to satisfy an itch, and when his hand reappeared, he was clutching a paper flower, bright pink, with floppy petals and a rubbery green stem. The little man stared at it as if in astonishment, and then he made a gesture of helplessness and flung it blindly over his shoulder.

"Well?" he said at last, facing the young man and folding his arms over his chest. "I'm not granting any *three* wishes today. Only this one. Do you or don't you?"

The young man raised the hatbox in his arms; if he could have watched himself at that moment, he would have seen the helplessness of the gesture, the way he gave himself away. "Is it near where the incubators are?"

Against his palm, which held the hatbox close to his chest, he felt a sudden flutter, as if what was inside could sense his excitement, sense that they were near their destination. It was the same rolling flutter, a mouse under a handkerchief, that he'd felt under Sylvie's tight belly. He had lain there next to her in the dark, his head on the soft indentation below her shoulder, his gaze trained through the bars of the fire escape into the sky, which was laboriously dripping a summer-night rain.

The little man cocked his head. "The babies? Are you asking me about the *babies?*" He seemed to be considering something.

At last he stuck out a hand. "Same price," he said.

The young man reached into his pocket and fished out a nickel. He held it out and the little man snatched it from his fingers, leaping away at a sprint. "Hurry!" the little man called back. "Going to be late!"

"Wait!" The young man's protest flew from his mouth. "Wait!" And then, as he saw his escort begin to disappear into the crowd, he, too, started to run.

They flew together down innumerable, twisting streets strung with pink-and-white flags, down alleyways paved with rounded gray-blue stones, slippery and slick. The little man's strange laughter bounced ahead of them like the sun's reflection dancing from the back of a gold watch, skimming the surface of the world. Just ahead of him, his laughing, wheezing evader dodged the crowds, the flocks of offended ladies, the pools of surprised, excited children, his ugly head down like a ram's grizzled horn.

And then they stopped, at last, before the door of a theater, a long line of patrons snaking out from the entrance.

The young man drew up and stopped, breathing hard, and bent over to catch his breath. He saw that he had dented part of the hatbox as he'd gripped it close. A wave of nausea spread over him; it made him almost ill that he might have borne down on one of the child's tiny limbs and squashed it.

"Here we are," said the little man cheerfully, pointing. "Babies—and a *babe* . . ."

But the young man ignored him. He looked up. Next to the theater, where an advertisement for Caroline Day's fan-dancing act filled the marquee, was a low white building shaped like a U; in the center of the U, facing the street, was a tree-filled courtyard occupied by two storks and a tall fountain like a beaker, spewing twin plumes of water, one tinged pink, the other blue. The letters of the exhibit were woven into an iron banner that spanned the courtyard between the two white wings: BABY INCUBATORS, the banner read. And beneath, ALL THE WORLD LOVES A BABY.

He took a deep breath and felt from within the hatbox what he thought was a tiny, answering sigh. He was pleased, a parent's first, astonished pride; they had done this together, *he and his son*. They were here.

T W O

St. Louis watched the young man climb the steps of the incubator exhibit—the baby house, as he called it. The man—though he was more of a boy, really—paused at the broad top step before the door; St. Louis could still see his chest rising and falling from the exertion of their run through the fairgrounds.

What business could that boy have in the baby house? St. Louis sat down on a bench across the street from the Lido, where he could watch the customers lining up for his cousin Caroline's next show and keep an eye on the young man at the same time. He wasn't sure what made this young man and his hatbox so interesting, but his behavior—furtive, exhausted, urgent—excited St. Louis's curiosity. What did he have in that hatbox, anyway?

St. Louis took the white mouse out of his pocket and set it down on the ground under the bench. It dove into the inviting opening of an overturned sack of popcorn. St. Louis had liberated a number of these white mice from the tent of the snake charmer, who kept them in a box for his snakes to eat. St. Louis didn't like the man—he'd seen him raise his hand once and strike the cringing, buxom girl who performed as his assistant. Ever since, St. Louis had gone by the snake charmer's tent almost every day and helped himself to a handful of the mice, which he then set free in auspicious spots in the fairgrounds.

The men standing in line at the Lido shoved one another with mock aggression; the women tittered behind their hands. St. Louis leaned over and unlaced his shoes; his feet hurt. He wasn't used to running like that anymore. It was the sort of stunt he'd pulled when he was younger, the sort of thing he didn't seem to have much energy for these days. One of his favorite tricks as a kid had been to pretend that one of his own hands had become possessed and was trying to strangle him. He did a very convincing performance of this. Children found it hilariously funny, but he could reduce certain adults to tears of laughter with the act, too. Caro herself was completely helpless whenever he started on it, and even some of the persistent men who were dangerously disappointed to discover that St. Louis would not offer them a personal introduction to Caro, no matter how many bills they folded up and tried to tuck into St. Louis's coat pocket, had been known to relent, smiling, when St. Louis fell to the ground, struggling and gagging and cursing.

What had made him do it, anyway, forcing the kid to run like that? Why had he even bothered him in the first place? God knows he didn't need the kid's nickel. It was something about how lost he'd looked, St. Louis thought, as if he were sleepwalking and needed to be woken up before he fell over a cliff.

But it was boredom, too, that had driven him to such a pointless display. Ever since the fair had opened a few weeks before, he'd found himself unaccountably bored by the crowds that came to see Caro and her fan dance. He didn't care about the money she made, money she had always shared freely with him—first formally, for his familial services as her protector, and then eventually just because that was their arrangement, St. Louis keeping watch over Caro, and Caro giving St. Louis his fragile sense of belonging in the world. "What would I do for intelligent conversation without you?" she asked him, joking, pressing bills into his hands. But he didn't want the money; he'd never really been able to think of what to spend it on, anyway. He'd bought a lot of pointless presents for people over the years—a canary for a blind pianist at a rooftop restaurant in Brooklyn, a foolish mink stole for the beautiful four-year-old daughter of a postman in Hoboken, a fleet of red bicycles for the children at an orphanage in Philadelphia—random acts of benevolence that now struck him as pathetic. And he was tired all the time, he told Caro. "I'm getting too old to do this," he'd complained to her on the train to Chicago. "I'm forty-four years old. I want . . . "

But he never could decide what it was that he wanted.

"You want a steak dinner." Caro hoped to soothe him. "You want a pet dog? A boat? A sailboat would be nice, on Lake Michigan."

But it wasn't any of those things. Recently he'd been aware of a vague but piercing sense of unhappiness, as though he was about to lose something he loved.

Massaging his heel, St. Louis turned his attention away from the restless crowds waiting before the Lido and back to the baby house; the young man still stood there uncertainly, the hatbox in his hands. In the courtyard, the storks paced delicately through their shallow lagoon, fastidiously lifting their feet free of the water after each step; under the climbing sun, their white feathers glowed. The fair's strangely shaped buildings and its often eccentric residents—men, women, and beasts—sometimes made St. Louis remember the flat, endless Illinois plains he and Caro had seen from the train on their way to Chicago, acres of corn and soybeans that stretched away into the distance, nothing against the horizon except the long, final seam of sky meeting earth. When he'd seen them for the first time, those fields had filled him with despair; it was as if nothing would ever happen again. But now he found the thought of them reassuring; planted against the flat, empty line of that horizon, even a small man, a man of no physical consequence, would stand out.

The fairgrounds, on the other hand, had unnerved him from the start. It was as if a subtle but significant shift had taken place in the world while his back was turned. Still, it was only the future—of architecture and everything else, he supposed— glimpsed through the clouds of the present. The fair's buildings were square and abrupt, with flat surfaces like Aztec temples, embellished with fins and friezes and pylons that hung on to the walls and roofs like afterthoughts. Or the structures were round and squat, inverted bowls painted in bold oranges and blues, black, and yellow. St. Louis had read the critics' initial responses, and he thought he could detect in the praises of the admirers a note of false witness. No one could really want the future to look like this, could they? How was a person to get his bearings in a world that looked like this?

In the weeks before the fair had opened, balmy spring days while the site was in the last stages of frenzied preparation, St. Louis had liked watching the construction of this foreign universe. He didn't have much to do: Caro was enjoying a swank hotel room in downtown Chicago before moving to her finished rooms in the Streets of Paris over a shoe shop near the Lido (St. Louis always arranged to have Caro's private quarters out of sight of the theater, to put some distance between occasionally overardent fans and Caro herself, but both of them liked to be housed at the fairgrounds; in the past, they'd never grown tired of seeing all there was to see). And because the baby house was next door to the Lido, where, as Caro's business manager, he felt he had a duty to oversee final preparations, he'd watched its construction especially carefully. The fair's architects had used wood for hardly anything. Instead, welders with their torches came in ranks, ten abreast, and fastened huge pieces of sheet metal to steel web-and-timber skeletons; buildings went up fast that way. He'd been hanging around the day the sign for the baby house was installed and had stayed to watch as it was swung into place over the courtyard one windy afternoon, the word BABIES tilting dangerously before it was righted. Over the next few days, he'd seen palm trees and potted hibiscus and bougainvillea and rolled yards of sod hauled in, and one day he saw the two storks—like giant, ugly ballerinas—unloaded from two crates the size of wardrobes and freed into the fenced courtyard. They'd been drugged for the trip, perhaps; one of them fell down on its spindly legs upon reaching the bright green grass. St. Louis had watched, alarmed, as the creature fell into the lagoon, struggled upright, and finally heaved itself back to dry land. St. Louis had looked around for someone to blame—he'd *hated* seeing that; why had he stayed to watch?—but the driver of the truck had gone inside the baby house.

Ten days before the fair opened, Caro had told him to take a few days off entirely. She had a friend in Chicago who'd look after her, she said, and she gave him two hundred dollars, an absurd amount. "Don't spend it all in one place," she told him. "I'll see you next week."

St. Louis had been glad not to have to play bodyguard to Caro for a few days; his usual job was to threaten the fellows who invariably came around after her show and wanted to buy her a drink. They often got into fights with one another, and though St. Louis couldn't really take on anybody in contests of strength—no one was much afraid of an ugly little man, almost a dwarf, as he thought of himself—he was skilled at jollying disappointed suitors out of their bad tempers. He told them Caro was actually hideously ugly. "She wears a mask over her face, see," he'd say, "and then at night, when she takes it off—" and here he would contort his face into grotesquely comic expressions, inverting his eyelids and rolling his eyes back in his head and baring his teeth. "But what a body, no?" he'd add, shaking his head in mock regret.

He hadn't really minded a few days with nothing particular to do. He had a feeling Caro wanted him out of the way while she had a forty-eight-hour love affair with some man; she never liked having St. Louis around when she enjoyed herself in this way. It was the family connection, he supposed.

But he hadn't really felt like leaving Chicago; where would he go, anyway? Instead, he'd hung around the fairgrounds, watching the final preparations. One day, there'd be an empty street laid out with string and chalk lines. The next day, storefronts were propped up, window boxes were filled with flowers, floors and walls were laid in single sheets, everything falling into place and raising clouds of dust. Teams of masons in blue aprons came through with troughs of cement. Painters in loose-fitting white overalls, with rags tied around their throats, hung suspended from rooflines and descended like snowy spiders along the faces of buildings, rappelling down the walls on springy feet, leaving bright washes of desert color—orange, turquoise, mustard—in their wakes. Everywhere there was industry and noise.

The theatrical light shows that were to dazzle so many spectators at the fair that summer were also rehearsed in those last days before the gates opened, and St. Louis would take a cigar and a beer and lie in the soft darkness in one of the paddle-boats in the lagoon to watch the beams of colored light flick on and off over his head, sweeping crazily over the lagoon. St. Louis also stood in front of the huge Western Union Panel, with its beautiful, richly colored map of the eastern United States, puzzling over the mysteries of the fair's electrical genesis. One night, one of the engineers explained to him how the lights worked: every night, from the astronomical observatories at Harvard, Allegheny College, the University of Illinois, and Yerkes at Lake Geneva, Wisconsin—their domes seen on the map at the fair as pinpricks of light—signals from the star Arcturus were received and trapped and in turn flashed to the panel on display in Chicago. As the fourth and last line of light—from the Yerkes observatory—darted across the face of the panel, the darkness hanging over the fairgrounds be-came light, and multicolored sweepers set to tilting over the la-goon, shards of color reflected in the platinum waters of Lake Michigan like broken glass.

"A million flying arrows of loveliness," intoned a voice over the loudspeaker, rehearsing, and the eyes of workmen leaving the fairgrounds for the night rolled obediently upward, heads on necks tilted back. Standing shoulder to shoulder with the delivery people and the masons and carpenters and welders and painters, St. Louis could see for himself how lovely it was. But it made him wary, too; he thought he recognized it for a chimera, some kind of trick. He himself had a repertoire of modest displays of sleight of hand—he'd never cared enough about it to get really good, but he could astonish drunks cer-tainly, which was fun, and even sober bartenders from time to time. He could do Penny through the Elbow, for instance, in which an ordinary penny appears to disappear into your arm, except that you have actually dropped it down your collar. Or the Dance of the Single Veil, which gave the effect of a handkerchief wriggling and moving about on its own. Or the Hanky-Panky Coin Vanish, for which you needed a secret rubber band. St. Louis thought he was familiar with the crude underpinnings of magic—his first magic book had explained about patter, for instance, the effect of distracting an audience: "I learned this trick while I was traveling in Hindustan, where I met a fakir," you were supposed to say. "Only he wasn't a real fakir—he was a fake fakir." So St. Louis recognized a setup. And at one level, he thought, the Century of Progress was one big setup.

He had to acknowledge, though, that there had been changes in the world since 1893, when Chicago's last world's fair, the Columbian Expo, had been held along Lake Michigan's shoreline. He hadn't been there for that fair; he and Caro were only babies then. But for a man with no money and what he thought of as a liquid store of possessions, he kept track of the country's economic fortunes. The rewards of thievery—even petty, amusing thievery such as he practiced occasionally for lack of anything better to do—suffered these days, along with everything else, though with less consequence, of course. He couldn't pick pockets when pockets were empty, after all, and he was moved at the sight of breadlines full of desperate men out of work. He'd bought strangers more bowls of Brunswick stew than he could count by now. Fortunately, he considered, there were always customers in Caro's line of work. It was as if no one, no matter how destitute, could do without the sight of Caro dancing behind her fans. The clientele for her shows had even risen a notch or two since things had gotten bad all around, as if the national financial crisis gave slumming a fashionable edge for men and women who, without their accustomed high-class luxuries, could accord Caro and her fan-dancing act a curious new status. But the new crowds were not as attentive as the old ones, he'd observed: They were less hushed and respectful, almost hysterically gay. They had the desperation of those accustomed to happiness who now found the world they knew crumbling at their feet. Still, St. Louis thought, though everything might fall away, there would be his cousin Caro, revealed in the wreckage, rising like Venus on the half shell, hope for a starving nation.

But even if people were poor in 1933—or still poor, anyway—when you go from a world where everybody gets around on horseback or in a carriage, or by streetcar or excursion boat, to a world where people can get in their own Ford automobiles or Studebakers or Rocknes without giving it a second thought, that's change, St. Louis had to admit. An open letter from Henry Ford in the paper the other day had declared, "We did not invent the eight-cylinder car. What we did was make it possible for the average family to own one." That was true enough, St. Louis conceded. Yet did change always mean progress? Though Roosevelt, of whom he approved, was now in office, and Prohibition was over (he approved of that, too), he thought that few people were any more content now than they'd been forty years before, in 1893, when the bottom fell out of the wheat market and farmers failed and fortunes collapsed at the board of trade. The same specter of financial ruin—the stock exchange's plummeting collapse in a humid October 1929, men leaping from office buildings in their shirtsleeves—hung over the country now as then. Rioting farmers in Iowa resisted foreclosure when their mortgages fell unavoidably into default. Thousands were without jobs. The gold standard had been abandoned. The commodity price of beef in Chicago had dropped 13 percent, and cattle on the hoof by only a little less. That spring, banks across the country had closed for two days in an unprecedented "banking holiday."

Even the great Babe Ruth had taken a ten-thousand-dollar pay cut last year without complaint.

But where the fair of 1893, with its pristine and classical architecture, had been known as the White City of the Unsalted Sea, this summer's Century of Progress, as the organizers called it, was to be crazy for color, St. Louis saw — crazy for light, for movement, for the hand's being quicker than the eye, for things no one could understand anymore by just looking at them. The people he would see this summer would look humble to him, he knew — eager to be pleased by what they saw, but often confused, too, and perhaps ashamed of their confusion. Wandering around the fairgrounds in the last days of May before the gates opened, he'd thought he could sense this intention on the part of the fair's organizers — a kind of relentlessness. People had to be *made* to believe. They had to feel their smallness, in a way, their ignorance, in order to desire the future, to need it, to believe they would be saved by what the future could offer. They had to want, unequivocally, even desperately, what the future offered — bigger and sleeker cars, freezers and refrigerators in every kitchen, airplane travel, superheterodyne radios, Technicolor movies, buildings taller than Chicago's Wrigley Tower or New York's Empire State Building. They had to be wooed and won by the light and the razzle-dazzle, and they had to yearn to jump off blindly into the swift currents of the future, even if they didn't know where the river would lead them.

The doors of the Lido opened finally, and the restless lines of waiting people standing in the street in front of St.

Louis began to disappear inside. St. Louis moved his cigar from one corner of his mouth to the other, let go of his right foot, and picked up his left to rub his toes. The boy and his hatbox were still there on the steps of the baby house. The boy had sat down now on the top step, the hatbox on his lap; he seemed to be waiting for something.

St. Louis thought it was funny, in a way, that Caro's act had ended up next to the incubator-baby exhibit. Surely, he had told Caro, someone—some newspaper reporter—would point out the irony of it when the fair opened. What fool had decided to make those innocent babies and a scandalizing fan dancer bunk mates? In city after city, there was always some delegation of prim, appalled matrons and their shamefaced husbands aiming to take down Caroline Day. Chicago would be no different, St. Louis suspected, and Caro's detractors would no doubt find her proximity to a nursery full of children especially outrageous.

But St. Louis was drawn to the baby house, all the same.

One day, a week before the fair opened, he saw an ambulance pull up to the curb in front of the baby house. A grave-looking man with a dark mustache and a black coat got out, accompanied by one of the ugliest women St. Louis had ever seen. This was the great Dr. Hoffman himself? St. Louis had heard of him on Coney Island, where Caro had performed and where the doctor ran his Infantorium year-round on the board-walk. St. Louis was surprised by how young Hoffman looked; he'd expected him to be older. In the back of the ambulance were the incubator boxes, shiny as polished stovepipe. St. Louis had wandered over to watch the unloading. Neither Hoffman nor the ugly nurse—he supposed she was a nurse—gave him a second look; they bustled into the building right away behind the procession of incubators rolled in on tiny wheels. But a car had pulled up behind the ambulance a few minutes later, and a group of plump, cheerful-looking young women had climbed out, extending legs in pale hose to the sidewalk and handing their babies to one another—these would have been the wet nurses, St. Louis guessed. He had caught the eye of one and winked, and she'd given him a grin. Women often liked him; that he was short made him seem unthreatening, perhaps. He was aware of playing this to his advantage in some ways. A full-grown man could not cavort, for instance, without looking insane, but St. Louis, because he was small, because he was funny to look at, could contrive a variety of physical poses that were seen as endearing. He could box at the air and make people laugh. He could don a pair of eyeglasses and evoke a studious child. (For this purpose he kept a pair of spectacles on hand.) By those who came to know him, he was frequently taken for a confessor, perhaps *because* he was not a beauty. "You just have one of those faces," Caro told him. "People like to tell you the most awful things."

On his sixth birthday Caro herself had told him the story of his birth. They'd been sitting on the hillside in back of the barn on Caro's family's farm in Pharaoh, Virginia. Caro, who was eight at the time, had lain on her stomach, lining up on the grass the little crowns of thorns that fell from the tulip poplar tree planted at the north corner of the barn.

"You came two months before anyone expected you," she told him, obliging him with what scant details she knew of his past. "You were puny as a skunk. They thought you'd die."

From Caro's mother, Irene—his own mother's oldest sister, who'd raised him after his mother's disappearance—he learned other grudging details. After falling in love with the man who became her husband—the bear trainer for a small circus that came through Richmond one summer—his mother had become the retinue's seamstress, sewing costumes and tents and doing general mending for the carnies and their families. Her husband and his bear would wrestle for the crowds, and men would spend fifty cents for the chance to pin the beast. But the bear trainer had disappeared long before St. Louis would have been conceived, Caro had told him; his aunt, when St. Louis asked about this detail in puzzlement, had frowned. "Some things it's better not to know," Irene had said, sighing. "Your mother always had great spirit, St. Louis, but perhaps she didn't always choose her life's companions wisely."

Still, Caro said he ought to go ahead and think of the bear trainer as his father anyway. "All your life, when people ask you what your father did for a living, you'll be able to say he wrestled grizzly bears." This, too, had been good for a laugh, St. Louis had discovered, because to imagine any relative of St. Louis's in the ring with a bear was to conjure up David and Goliath. The disadvantage was good for sympathy.

The circus had been summering in the city of St. Louis at the time of his birth—this accounted for his first name, his aunt had told him. But he would never know the origin of his last name, Percy—whether the name was perhaps his father's (first or last, he'd never know) or just something that had struck his mother. He had no memory of the scrappy, doomed, familial group into which he had been born, a fact that troubled him. Later on, he could imagine too well what his mother's life had been like: feeding the single elephant, painting the equipment, plaiting the ponies' manes, tying knots where they were needed. This much he'd seen for himself at carnivals and amusement parks around the country, following Caro from engagement to engagement. This much, he sometimes thought, and a lot more—a lot of ugliness, man to man, and man to woman, and woman to man.

His mother had become a mystery herself, disappearing from St. Louis's life when he was just shy of his second birthday. She brought him to her sister and brother-in-law in Virginia, with promises that she'd return for him when she had some money and "respectability." But she never did reappear, and after a while the only time St. Louis ever thought of her was when he went and looked at the somber studio portrait of the three sisters—his own mother, Ella; his aunt Irene; and their sister, Nell, who died from tuberculosis when she was sixteen. His mother had been a pretty, dark-eyed girl with a slightly lopsided face. In the photograph she was squinting as if sizing up some distant route of escape, a pinhole of opportunity far away in the blue clouds that held steady over the Blue Ridge Mountains of her childhood in a pose of infinite and sovereign patience.

But unlike his father, who seemed so ephemeral as never to have existed at all, St. Louis's mother had not wished him to forget her entirely or to think the worst of her for abandoning him. In an illiterate and incomprehensible letter full of inane benedictions, mailed to him from somewhere in New Mexico when he was seven, she had wished for him all the joy and happiness to be found in life.

Irene had received her sister's child with tender but—as it was her nature to be economical, even in emotional matters, St. Louis learned—reserved kindness. He viewed himself as an ugly man, and he supposed that he had been an ugly child, even at two. But he also saw that people tended to smile on him, rather than look away in disgust, the way they turned away from a particular man in Pharaoh who ran the grain mill and had his face burned in a bad fire. St. Louis's aunt told him that his chief advantage was the color of his eyes, a meltingly rich brown that she said reminded her of chocolate and would no doubt help people dispose themselves kindly toward him.

But he did not ever become handsome. He stopped growing at under five feet, and his face always looked wrong when he stared at himself in the mirror—as though his head and his body did not belong together. In his aunt's copy of Hans Christian Andersen's fairy tales, he found an illustration by Arthur Szyk of the vain girl with the beautiful red shoes that danced her away into the pauper's graveyard and refused to let her rest until her feet were chopped off by the executioner. Something about the child's expression in the drawing in the book—the eyes too large and baleful, the pinched chin, the forehead high and broad and glistening, as if swelling with a tumor—reminded him of himself, and he stared at the awful child. Eventually she had repented and become humble and pious. Yet it seemed no reward at all to him to end as this child did—her heart so filled with sunshine, peace, and joy that it breaks while she sits on her bench at church, her crutches by her side.

"*Was* it a dwarf, do you think?" St. Louis overheard Irene ask her husband as they got ready for bed one night. St. Louis lay quietly in his bed in the next room, listening to the elastic choir of tree frogs singing in the darkening meadow below the house and to the soft conversation of his aunt and uncle.

Warren grunted; St. Louis heard the bedsprings protest as Warren sat down and rolled onto his side, hauling a corner of the sheet with him. "Knowing your sister," he heard Warren answer at last, "it was probably *some* kind of freak."

He'd had to ask his aunt about his size once, a long time ago. He'd been ten, small for his age, though well devel-

oped, almost barrel-chested. One warm fall afternoon, he'd
stood on the lowest step by the kitchen door, fidgeting while
his aunt sat behind him and tried to keep him quiet between
her thighs as she trimmed his hair. Clouds the color of bruises
had moved along the edge of the mountains in the distance,
and an occasional roll of thunder melted into the hot air.
Warren had done the second mowing in the pasture below; the
hay lay in sagging rows. Fat chickens the color of bright pen-
nies fussed around St. Louis's feet, pecking at his clipped hair,
the soft brown tufts tumbling over the dirt and into the dark,
stinking places under the boxwoods.

"Am I a . . . dwarf?" The question had been forming in his
mind for such a long time that when he heard the sound of his
own voice framing the words, he waited for something to happen finally—for the old apple tree to split in half down its
fork, rain to loosen from the sky overhead, anything. But after
a moment in which nothing happened, he felt his aunt shake
her head behind him. "No, I don't believe so."

He waited a minute. "Almost a dwarf?"

Another pause. "Perhaps," she conceded, and her hands
stopped for a second. Then, snip, snip: his hair fell around him
into the grass again. The one-eyed chicken lunged for it and
missed; she was thinner every day since losing her eye to the
rooster. He bent over quickly to cup a passing grasshopper,
dangled it before the chicken, and watched her aim sideways
for it and finally snatch it with her beak.

"OK," he said, and he put his hand up to his new, tender
hairline as his aunt stood, brushing off her apron.

Not a dwarf then. Almost a dwarf.

A boy named for a city, not a saint, but that was his name
anyway, the name they all called him. St. Louis. Almost-a-
dwarf St. Louis.

The day the letter had come from his mother, St. Louis had been sitting on the back steps of the farmhouse again, a kitten in his lap and a glass of lemonade on the step beside him. Irene touched his head lightly with her fingertips, sat down beside him, and handed him the letter. She did not ask him to read it to her, and St. Louis did not offer. He folded it when he was finished and put it in his pocket. He stared at the ground, his heart caroming against his ribs, his eyes following the desperate struggles of a beetle hauling a sugar crystal, which had fallen from his lemonade spoon, up the steep ascent of a blade of grass.

Irene watched the boy with what he knew was pity. St. Louis could sense her worried expression, even though he did not look up directly into her face. She began to open her mouth to say something but discovered, he surmised, that she had no words of comfort for him. And so she said nothing at all, moving quietly away from him at last, going back into the house out of the still, hot, late-afternoon air.

For a long time St. Louis didn't move from his spot on the lowest porch step. He held the black kitten close to his chest. Eventually, bored in the anxious vice of the boy's hands, it bit his thumb lightly in frustration, and he let it go. When the sun began to go down and he was called in to supper, he stood up; his knees and backside were stiff and sore. He looked briefly up into an evening sky that poured down an abundance of stars and then out across the rolling Virginia meadows that lifted like waves in the sea, shifting levels of lightning bugs twinkling in the dark. And then he turned around and went inside to eat. There didn't seem anything else to do.

But Caro became his coach in this matter, as in so many ways. She liked to dress up in her mother's discarded clothes and made St. Louis play with her. He wanted to be the hero, of

course, and begged for his uncle's smart army uniform. But
Caro shook her head. "You have to be the magician," she said,
winding turbans around his head instead, or "You have to be
Rumpelstiltskin," or "You have to be the Billy Goat Gruff." And
he found that she was right. He was good at these roles — good
at hooked noses, which he could fashion out of a segment of an
egg carton, whittled into a beak with his knife. He was good at
cloven hooves, which he could suggest by prancing. He was
good at hunchbacks and wizards and sorcerers. Caro painted
red circles on his cheeks and called him a clown. In winter she
broke off icicles from the eaves of the porch and showed him
how to stand on the porch swing, murmuring incantations, a
tablecloth pinned over his shoulders. In spring she gave him
antlers of forsythia. In summer she made him wreaths of dan-
delions, and he knelt in the tall grass and roared.

Together they looked up *dwarf* in the dictionary. "Dwarf
alder, dwarf chestnut, dwarf cornel . . ." she read aloud.

"Those are all just short bushes," he said, pained.

"But look." She stopped, her finger on the page. "Dwarf
elder."

He started to protest. "That's just a short elder tree —"

"But listen to how it sounds," she said. "Dwarf *elder*." She
snapped the book closed, stood up, and touched his shoulder
with a wooden spoon. "Dwarf *elder*. Like a wise man. That's
you."

St. Louis looked down at the ground.

"Rise up," she said. "Rise up, dwarf elder."

And when he did stand at last and look up at her, she was
not laughing at him. He could feel tears in his own eyes, but
her expression was kind. "All clowns are sad," she told him.
"That's why we love them."

• • •

St. Louis saw that Irene Day was careful to spread her affections evenly between himself and Caro, but he suspected that he was the easier of the children to live with, in a way — Caro was wild and clever and intimidating, even as a child. St. Louis, on the other hand, had a sense of humor and careful, quiet motions that made him useful with the farm animals. When Irene took the children's hands to walk with them into the brick Baptist church high on the hill above Pharaoh, he enjoyed the feeling of her calm grip, soft and warm, and he was glad he could make her the gift of returning her affection, for he felt grateful to her. Caro could rarely bear to hold hands with anyone.

The Days could not have foreseen, any more than St. Louis himself, that their daughter would one day deprive them first of herself and then of St. Louis, too, who knew he would not live a week without Caro — their affection for each other was genuine and deep, though sometimes St. Louis thought Caro needed him the way a host needs a parasite. But he had seen Irene watching him and Caro play from a window in the dim front parlor, Caro dancing like a gypsy in the high grass of the meadow, and St. Louis — considerably shorter than his cousin — barreling through the brown and silver fronds behind her, leaving a wide, rough trough in his wake. At the end of an afternoon of playing, St. Louis would be red-faced and slick with perspiration; but Caro could run for miles and never break a sweat.

"You're not a human being," St. Louis would tell her, throwing himself down on the porch swing. "I need to pinch you."

The fact that Caro, who began as a milliner's model, discovered she had a talent for dancing — and in the nude, no less — did not surprise St. Louis.

But it came as a shock to her parents.

Irene and Warren Day did not have much, but what they did
have they shared generously with their nephew—in the manner of impoverished but kindly figures in fairy tales, St. Louis
recognized. They sold field crops, milk from their small herd of
dairy cows, and eggs. Their living had been a modest one, with
one exception. Their property had one advantage, a feature
that set it apart from the neighboring farms and gave it a certain distinction. It had a spring.

Warren, who had been an officer in the Spanish-American
War, wouldn't have risked the capital trying to turn his spring
into the sort of watering resort popular over in West Virginia,
where other natural lithia waters were being touted as the antidote to a long list of ailments and were attracting swarms of
pilgrims eager to take the cure. Warren was not a risk-taking
man. But he was not without shrewdness, and he had looked
for a special market for his springwater. Purely by accident—
he happened to break an ankle getting off the train in Richmond
one day on business and was tended to by a fellow passenger,
the doctor for the Eastern State Penitentiary in Philadelphia—
Warren began marketing his lithia water to area jails. Soon he
had a corner on physicians to much of the convict population
in Virginia, as well as a small clientele in and around Pharaoh
itself.

When St. Louis was young, he had drunk quantities of this
water, standing secretly by the spring, rigid with expectation,
just before dawn or after dark—hours he felt were better for
magic. He drank until he thought he would burst, willing his
life to change, willing himself to be tall, to be handsome, to be
fortunate, to be loved, willing something wonderful to happen.
But it had never made any difference, as far as he could see—
except, maybe, for the part about being loved, for Caro did love
him. If St. Louis was sure of anything, he was sure of that.

Irene had died three years ago, in the fall of 1930. Caro and St. Louis had arrived in Pharaoh from New York some hours after the fact, as though Caro had timed their homecoming to miss the worst of it. St. Louis alone knew that Caro had delayed unnecessarily, busying herself with various errands, deciding to wash her hair at the last minute, missing one train and then another; yet he also understood that it had been fear, not cruelty, that had kept her away.

They did not stay even three full days. The morning after Irene's funeral, a humid, ashen August day, St. Louis had stepped out onto the porch of the old farmhouse, troubled by the silence that lay thickly in the rooms. It was as if, all these years, only his aunt's presence had stood between them and this creeping decay, the filthy nature of a neglected world. Irene had always worn an apron, he remembered.

Caro had a radio playing in a back bedroom as she dressed for the train. The sound was small and incidental, far away, as if St. Louis might be imagining it or as if it were an insect troubling the air around his head. Stepping outside onto the porch, allowing the split screen doors to fall closed behind him with the sharp report of dead wood, he'd seen his uncle standing at the top of the hill just past the barn, a long, forked stick in his hand, his hand shielding his eyes against the bright slant of morning light. St. Louis walked up the hill, past the abandoned chicken coop thick with cottony spiderwebs, past the barn, part of its roof sliding ominously toward the ground.

He came up beside Warren and looked out over the fields, the distant, steaming hills drifting with haze, the erratic lacing of trees. The meadow below them was studded with sharp thistles. Warren did not seem to notice St. Louis standing there beside him.

St. Louis had cleared his throat. "Don't keep the cows anymore?"

Warren shook his head.

St. Louis let his eyes flicker over the fallow fields. "Grow beans this year? Sweet potatoes?"

Again, Warren shook his head. His mouth seemed to flatten out as he stared ahead of him.

St. Louis frowned, ran a hand through his hair. Then he brightened. He turned to Warren, reached up to touch his uncle's shoulder. "Let's walk down to the spring," he proposed. "There's time before our train. I haven't had a drink of water that good in years."

And suddenly he could taste it, could feel rising in his heart the same flag of hope that had risen each time he had knelt at the stone font and filled his cup. Anything was possible.

But Warren turned to him, his eyes dead, his skin liver-colored and leathery. "It's dried up," he said. He glanced away, as if St. Louis did not matter to him anymore. "It might have saved Irene," he said, "but it's dried up." He waited. "It's been a terrible year," he said, his voice shaking.

St. Louis had felt the impact of this information in his chest, as though Warren had just shoved him with the heel of his palm. Warren squinted ahead, as though trying to fix in his eye some distant image. And then, with a motion that made St. Louis suddenly wary, he shifted his weight, like a fighter. He opened his mouth: "Does she take off everything?"

There was a buzzing beneath St. Louis's feet as though he'd stepped on a hive of bees, something dangerous concealed in the grass; he could feel the heat of his uncle's rage and pain pulsing off him in waves, making him smell sour. And the spring, he'd thought inconsequentially, the spring. The spring was dried up; the water he'd once imagined would make him whole had retreated to its secret core in the earth. St. Louis and his kind were simply not worth saving.

He raised his eyes to his uncle's face: *Don't think the worst of us. It's not a bad life.*

But Warren seemed far away, like a planet moving out coldly on the tether of its distant orbit, beyond reach.

Warren shrugged. "I just want to know," he said, "if she's a whore, too."

St. Louis looked down at his feet. "No," he said at last. "No, sir. Not a whore."

He and Caro had left an hour later. She had an engagement dancing in Philly.

From his seat on the bench across the street from the Lido, St. Louis sat forward. The boy with the hatbox had stood up finally and stepped aside to let a crowd of people out the doors, mostly women, mopping at their cheeks with handkerchiefs. St. Louis understood their discomfort. He himself had found the sight of those babies troubling. And Caro said she wouldn't go in there for all the tea in China. "Who wants to see a thing like *that?*" she'd said in genuine horror.

But St. Louis had gone to see one of the first shows. One morning he saw Alice Vernon—he'd learned her name in a matter of days—the ugly nurse whose flesh fell from her arms and chin like frozen waterfalls, who did her hair in two knots round as snake charmers' baskets at either side of her head, returning to the building with a basket of roses in her arms. Something about that gesture, the notion of providing roses for the babies, had made St. Louis want to go inside. He was, in fact, a little late for the first show, detained by a streak of luck at the poker table with the waiters from the Café de la Paix, who played every afternoon after the lunch rush. But he'd folded his hand at last after checking his pocket watch, run through the Streets of Paris, and given the ticket taker at the baby house a chit for Caro's show. (He often traded them for a meal and a drink or a cigar, just for the pleasure of striking a transaction with someone.)

When he stepped into the exhibition room at the nursery and squirmed his way to the front of the crowd, Alice Vernon was opening the door to one of the incubators. She extended her hand inside the box. Next to the baby, her massive arm looked like a giant's, like those two arms, nurse's and baby's, weren't the same thing at all and never would be.

The crowd that day was made up almost entirely of women and a few thin, bedraggled men—none of them very well off, St. Louis surmised, judging from their cheap, worn shoes and plain clothes, the dark circles under their eyes. They stood in a tight cluster, as if they might be surprised by something and needed to stay close together, behind the rope that separated them from the row of gleaming incubators with their silver pipes and intricate-looking valves. A low breathing noise filled the room, like the regular wheeze of a mechanical lung. Another nurse was explaining how the incubators worked.

Very gently, as the crowd watched, Alice Vernon turned one of the infants so that the onlookers, standing on tiptoe, could see its tiny, closed-up face.

And then, pulling from her own finger a huge diamond ring—paste, St. Louis determined at a glance—Alice Vernon turned and displayed it briefly to the audience, like a magician flashing an egg or a coin.

The women around St. Louis stood open-mouthed.

Leaning back inside the incubator, Alice Vernon slipped the ring over the wrist of the baby inside. It rode up the infant's arm and rested there, wildly, wrongly disproportionate.

The women in the audience moaned a little, but St. Louis had had enough.

It didn't seem right to him, not then, nor later, as he watched people line up, day after day, show after show, to go into the baby house. It didn't seem right, gawking at these babies, so tiny that a woman's ring could run up over their elbows. It had struck him uncomfortably, in fact, that the expressions of the women staring in at the infants had been not unlike those of the men who came to watch Caro dance, something grateful and pathetic coming over their faces as the ostrich feathers of her twin fans worked up and down, up and down, fanning the smoky blue air over Caro's breasts.

And this business of taking *money* from people who would come and stare at someone else's poor unfortunate baby, a child who didn't look big enough to put in a pot and boil—it bothered him. And then they'd turn around and go eat themselves a hot dog, or a bag of popcorn, or sit down before Madame Zenda and have their fortunes told! What were they doing here, these babies, these human beings, these *people?* What did these babies have in common with Captain Kelly, that maniac who dove off a 104-foot platform into a little tank of water? What did they have in common with armless wonder Martha Morris, or the microcephalics, or the Blue Man, who drank silver nitrate to dye his skin? St. Louis had seen all this and more at circuses across the country, at Coney Island, where he'd done a turn for a few summers as a night watchman for Dreamland, the biggest amusement park ever built. Every night he'd cross from Heaven to Hell on the sawdust roads of the amusement park and back again.

He'd seen all the tricks already from his days at Coney Island—the Siamese twins who had a fight onstage and split apart, tearing in half the corset that bound them at the rib cage. This had made him laugh, but it hadn't really surprised him. Nothing much surprised him anymore—not the wild man from Borneo, nor the Human Blockhead, who drove nails into his skull, nor Coney Island's bearded lady, poor soul, with her collection of tortoiseshell combs and her penchant for marshmallows, which she ate from paper sacks. Hidden behind a tent flap, St. Louis used to watch her respectfully, as a friend watches another friend grieve; she burrowed into the bag and devoured its contents, tears running into her chestnut beard.

For these people he felt pity, sometimes, and occasionally a sense of comradeship—after all, wasn't he his own kind of freak?—and from time to time a shocking, passionate hatred: Though "Sober Sir Edward" offered to pay one hundred dollars to anyone who could make him smile, St. Louis had never seen him smile, not once, not even when Sir Edward wasn't working but was sitting at the bar at Feltman's Hotel on West Fifth Street in New York, drinking himself into a thick stupor. *What's the matter with you?* St. Louis had fumed silently, cracking peanut shells between his fingers. He'd wanted, from ten bar stools away, to crash through the tables between them and take Sir Edward by the throat with both hands. *Smile, why don't you?* he wanted to say. *Can't you see how funny it is?*

No, these babies did not fall into the same category as these others, though Dr. Hoffman showed them at fairs and expositions, St. Louis knew: the Coney Island barkers under their sandwich boards paced up and down the boardwalks, calling to the crowds, "Don't pass the babies by!"

St. Louis stood up, crushing his cigar under his heel. The boy and his hatbox had stood up, but he still waited there uncertainly. What was the matter with him? If he wanted to go inside, why didn't he just open the door?

The storks in front of the baby house were restless, obsessively circling the little pond in the middle of their courtyard,
as if something might rise from its glassy surface. St. Louis
watched them. Something was wrong: the storks just kept walking their trammeled path, a desperate pacing. St. Louis felt a
pang of sorrow—for all the animals at the fair with iron chains
around their legs, for the babies with diamond rings on their
forearms, for all the damaged people he'd known. Nothing in
Chicago's Century of Progress could compare with the babies
inside that building, he thought. Because no one really knew—
not even Hoffman, he suspected—how they worked, how any
of us work, why some live and some die, what little spark of genius flares like a matchstick along the spine, ignites the seat of
the soul, and shoots up to tell the heart and brain to make the
body live. What, in the end, makes the heart beat, makes the
eyes open and close, makes the mouth murmur words?

The young man stood there—it had been nearly an hour
now, St. Louis saw, frowning, checking his watch—staring
down at the hatbox in his hands. As St. Louis stared at him, a
long, echoing silence seemed to drift down from the sky. St.
Louis felt a light chill, an odd sensation given the heat of the
day, run up his spine.

And then one of the storks, which had been standing still as
a statue near the far wall of the enclosure, began to run on its
spindly legs, its clipped wings cocked fiercely, toward the
young man hesitating by the door. St. Louis saw the boy start
in alarm. And then, as if in flight from the bird's strangely ag-
gressive assault—but there was a fence between them, wasn't
there?—the young man wrenched open the door and disappeared inside.

The stork stopped inches from the wrought iron gate, raised
one leg, sank its head into its breast, and closed its eyes.

St. Louis sat back down on the bench. He took a deep breath, a long inhalation, and closed his eyes; then he opened them again a second later to stare at the heavy doors of the incubator-baby show, where they had swung slowly closed with a final, inaudible click. Like an image retained against the prism of the eye, the shape of the young man, the hatbox under his arm, burned there a moment against the doors—the flaming silhouette through which circus performers make their exit—and then vanished.

The storks were circling and circling their pool. A band of acrobats came flying down the street past St. Louis, their checkered pantaloons billowing. A man with a monkey on his arm, the creature straining to stand on its hind legs and wringing its little hands, walked behind the acrobats. People dropped coins into the man's upturned hat. St. Louis looked up into the sky. The dirigible closed in overhead, hovering, casting a shadow in the shape of a bomb over the street below. St. Louis waited, holding his breath.

And then he sat bolt upright. A thought had pricked him, a needle breaking his skin.

The hatbox.

There was a baby in that hatbox.

THREE

"Well, it's not the first time we've had one come in like this, is it?" Dr. Leo Hoffman said. "Remember the—what was it? Apple crate?"

Alice Vernon looked at him reprovingly. "It was an onion box."

Dr. Hoffman watched her face move as she recalled the smell; how startling it had been to lift the lid and find a tiny baby inside, its head no bigger than a small orange, bedded down on crumpled paper and a bit of blanket. He should have remembered.

"It was an onion box, *not* an apple crate," Alice repeated, "and we never saw those parents at all. I don't think this one will be coming back, either. He looked done in."

Dr. Hoffman removed the stethoscope from his ears and sighed. "Then I suppose all we have left right now is our good faith that he will return."

Alice snorted. Dr. Hoffman knew Alice had a dim view overall of human nature. She had seen too many parents abandon their children to be persuaded of the nobility of the human heart, especially the adult human heart. She adored the babies. But she had no use for adults.

Dr. Hoffman frowned, gazing down at the newcomer to his nursery. Premature babies, this one so small Dr. Hoffman could have fit it inside his shoe, occasionally had this child's odd swarthiness. Dark, silky hair grew over the baby's temples and across his shoulders. Alice had settled him on his back in the incubator. His face, smaller than Dr. Hoffman's fist, worked in a series of grimaces, his eyes squeezed shut; he looked as though he wanted to cry but was distracted from the impulse over and over again by the startling presence of his own body, his arms flailing and flinging wide in a reflex, his legs kicking spasmodically, his tiny hands raking his cheek or ear. Dr. Hoffman reached in and turned the baby to lie on his stomach. Infants as small as this one were often uncomfortable on their backs, he'd noticed. He imagined they felt unstable that way, in danger of tumbling off the edge of the world. He watched the baby gather up his legs and drop instantly into sleep. For a moment, Dr. Hoffman was filled with pity. It looked like the narcotic sleep of someone who was begging for oblivion.

"He's exhausted," he said.

Alice looked down at the baby with him. "I say it's a miracle he's not dead." She stepped away, patting Dr. Hoffman on the shoulder as she went. "Well, he's all yours."

Dr. Hoffman raised his hand involuntarily to his mustache. It was a bad habit; he suspected it made him appear nervous, touching his face like that, and yet he didn't seem able to stop doing it. Sometimes he wanted to shave the thing off, despite what he thought of as its advantage of making him appear older and more dignified. He was often taken for a man in his thirties, though he would turn forty-five next March. He had the clear skin of childhood, as if he were strangely inexperienced in the world and had not yet been soiled by his encounter with it. (The wet nurses thought him handsome; they watched his eyes when they nursed the babies in his ward, but they never saw anything other than professional interest from him.) Though he could remember his father thoughtfully twirling his own mustache while he considered matters, Dr. Hoffman had been shocked nonetheless to see it appear in his own behavior sometime in his early forties. It was an errant defect, this bad habit—a knot or a whorl in a planed board that shows up stubbornly over time through layers of paint.

He stood by the incubator for a long while. He could tell a great deal just by looking at a baby and was always grateful when circumstances permitted such quiet inspection. He was amazed that a child so fragile—just under three pounds—should have survived the journey to the fair in a hatbox; he judged the infant to be thirty-two or thirty-three weeks along gestationally, though small for its age. Yet the parents, whoever they were, had done about as well as they could for the child, after all. He thought of the hatbox—what had the baby's father done with it? Suddenly the idea of it struck him almost comically as womblike, with its round sides and quilted satin cushioning. Better than an onion box, no doubt.

The baby, though dehydrated, had made it this far, and that was a good sign in and of itself. Dr. Hoffman appreciated it when a baby surprised him, surviving against the most astonishing odds. He'd read recently that an infant born in the United States at the beginning of the century was more likely to perish during its first year than an aviator who set out to take a plane up into the skies every day for a twelve-month period. Obviously, simply being small and fragile was the more dangerous enterprise of the two. Over one hundred thousand babies born every year died within the first four weeks of life as a result of what health authorities broadly termed congenital diseases: weakness or debility, prematurity, convulsions, marasmus, malformations, accidents, and injuries. There were half again as many stillbirths, a number Dr. Hoffman suspected was underreported, and the U.S. Census Bureau reported an alarming increase in the rate of death attributable to birth injury. But premature infants were especially predisposed to all manner of risk—intracranial hemorrhage, for instance, particularly around the seventh month of uterogestation, but also after birth as well. Such events, if they didn't kill the child outright, would certainly leave it deformed in some tragic way, a victim of spastic paralysis or imbecility or both. And then there were all the varieties of septic infection, not to mention asphyxia, atelectasis, pneumonia, convulsions, rickets, spasmophilia . . . Dr. Hoffman had observed over his years of treating babies that the will to live seemed unevenly doled out. Clearly some infants, and some adults as well, he supposed, possessed more stamina for survival than others. But still, there was really no telling what the future would bring for this baby, and he was, like all those who come before their time, poorly equipped to survive in the world. Nearly every organ, from his skin to his heart, was underdeveloped and immature and poorly functioning. So far, he was showing himself master of his domain, but Dr. Hoffman had seen babies who looked solid in the morning dead by suppertime, and he would take no bets on this child.

Watching this newcomer to his nursery, Dr. Hoffman found himself sadly amused, more than anything else. Here he was, his infants each costing him nearly $150 a day in overhead expenses—and of course the parents had no money for such extraordinary fees—here he was, still like a *common showman,* charging 25¢ a viewing to raise sufficient funds to cover his costs and divert whatever profits he could manage to research and equipment. Yet this little boy, with his narrow, angled head so typical of the premature infant, his gray-white fingers like minute, distended larvae, the dusky covering of hair over his body—this tiny creature so ill-fitted for survival had managed to make it through a long, hot morning in a hatbox at Chicago's world's fair. That it breathed on its own was nothing short of miraculous. Even as Dr. Hoffman watched, the infant's color seemed to improve under the steady influence of oxygen concentrations being blown gently into the incubator. And when Dr. Hoffman pressed his finger to the child's arm, he saw that the baby's capillary action had improved, too—blood leaped back up to the surface of the skin in an instant. He wished the child's father would return—for many reasons, but especially because he wanted to have some whole or citrated blood from the father for prophylactic injections, in case the child took a sudden turn.

What were the odds for this baby? In his student days at the Paris Maternité, Dr. Hoffman had learned the account of an infant weighing just 680 grams—1 pound 8 ounces—at birth. Though her circumstances could not have been less conducive to survival—the year was 1848, and no one knew anything about premature infants at the time—she had been kept alive in a chair near her family's open fireplace by regular, minute doses of cream and sherry. And he had read the reports from an anthropologist studying the Thonga, a South African tribe that allegedly cared for its early young by wrapping the infants in the leaves of the castor-oil plant, putting them in pots, and setting them out in the sun to bake. An astonishing number appeared to thrive under that prescription, if the anthropologist's stories were to be believed; Dr. Hoffman had his doubts.

Dr. Hoffman sighed and straightened his back, resting his palm briefly on the incubator's gleaming hood. The dry, sweet trace of oxygen lingered in the air, a scent to which he'd become so accustomed, since beginning the regular use of it in the incubators two years before, that ordinary air now seemed impoverished to him. There were twenty neonates with him in Chicago this year, mostly referred from the city's Sarah Morris Hospital by his friend Dr. Elliott Ludwig, with whom he had studied many years ago, who now ran the infant nursery there, one of only a handful in the entire country. Five of the twenty babies had been brought in during the first few days of the fair in Dr. Hoffman's own invention, the ambulance incubator. These were trips he was not eager to repeat, and he had told Dr. Ludwig as much. He and Alice had gone themselves to the designated households to fetch the infants—in some cases just hours after their birth—and Dr. Hoffman had found himself in the familiar but uncomfortable position of feeling utterly inadequate to the task of reassuring the parents. One mother—this was her first birth—had been crazed with grief and anxiety, and he had seen, even as he tried to be helpful, how austere and diffident his manner with her became in the face of her terror. Most mothers, he sensed, felt themselves at fault in some way when their infants arrived so early; and these women came to see this transaction with the doctor—this turning over of their babies—as a necessary punishment. *Remarkable*, he thought, *how many of us are so congenitally guilty.*

Still, he could guess that several of this summer's arrivals would find themselves orphans when it was time to leave the nursery. Some parents simply would not take their children back when the time came. He reminded himself again to ask Dr. Ludwig about adoptions; he had said something the other day about a woman from Chicago's Infant Aid Society being willing to help.

Now, with this new addition, there would be twenty-one babies in his nursery at the Century of Progress Exposition. This new arrival represented an unknown, and Dr. Hoffman was worried. For though he would not admit it, scarcely even to himself, he had wanted a perfect record this summer. Not one death.

Dr. Hoffman knew that his "attraction," as the fair board continued to refer to it, was second in earnings only to Caroline Day, the fan dancer; she was inarguably the fair's biggest and most popular show, but the babies were a close second. In Europe, when he had begun showing the preemies twenty years before, there had been reverence for his work, and he had been treated with deference and respect. Now some expos held on the Continent no longer invited him, only recently offended by the notion of showing live human beings to the public for a fee. Yet here in the United States, it was completely different. Here, people seemed to see Dr. Hoffman himself and his babies almost as freaks, and they were happy to attach a commercial value to the enterprise—newspaper accounts of his work were nearly always wrong, reporting babies at impossible weights of one pound or less, claiming that the babies' heads were no bigger than plums, that they could live days without sustenance of any kind.

He was baffled by this need to exaggerate. Wasn't the truth astonishing enough? Yet as he looked around this summer at the fair, this Century of Progress, as they called it, he understood that this decade was one of wild claims and promises, of staggering achievements and discoveries, of things bigger and better and easier and faster. This was the fair of superlatives. And so he felt particularly the pressure of his nursery this summer. Perhaps if he could have a 100 percent success rate with his babies this season, not a single mortality—perhaps if all these babies could be gathered for a reunion in the fair's second season next summer, whole and smiling and fatcheeked—then he would be free as he had never been before. He would not have to run his hospital next to naked ladies and fire-eaters and midget shows anymore. He and his babies could be where they belonged in fairs to come: in the halls of science.

This unusual marriage of medicine and carnival, which seemed to have become his career, had proved complicated in ways Dr. Hoffman could not have foreseen, though he did not blame himself for these complexities. Still, he was often troubled by the way his necessity for public support affected his decisions. There had been the matter of those quintuplets, for instance, this past spring. A newspaper publisher had contacted him personally, offering to charter an airplane and send him to Montana with a photographer and a reporter. But Dr. Hoffman had declined, citing his responsibility to his charges in Chicago. Later, though, talking it over with Dr. Ludwig, he confessed that he had not expected the quints to live. That suspicion—even more than the difficulties of getting oxygen and other supplies into the wilderness—had influenced his decision to stay in Chicago. "Imagine if they'd *all* died," he'd said to Dr. Ludwig. "I'd have a black mark on my forehead I'd never in a lifetime be rid of."

Late at night, though, when he scrutinized this attitude, he found something more than distasteful in it. *No physician likes to lose a patient*, he thought, *but what kind of doctor am I if I turn one away because I think his chances look poor?*

But there was plenty left to worry about here in his own nursery. He had screened the infants from Dr. Ludwig. They

had tacitly agreed that there was no point in taking unnecessary risks—even a three-and-a-half-pound baby looked small
to the general public and yet was considerably less likely to
succumb under Dr. Hoffman's care than one of two pounds or
less, though those did not often survive, in any case. But the
last five acquisitions, which Dr. Ludwig had urged him to take
for purposes of good feeling among Chicagoans, were smaller
and more sickly than Dr. Hoffman would have liked. And now
this latest arrival—it was a complete unknown. What sort of
conditions had it been born under? What diseases might the
mother be carrying? It wasn't unlikely that she was syphilitic.
What infections might the child himself be harboring? he wondered, peering through the glass doors at it.

He knew the road ahead for this small creature all too well,
how many things could go wrong. He worried chiefly about
cyanosis now, the most common symptom of inanition fever or
dehydration. Though the child had been kept warm, it had certainly been weak and dehydrated. Alice had given it a gavage
feeding of two cc's of breast milk—half a teaspoon—but she
reported that it had balked and fussed and stopped breathing
for a moment. "A strong enough cry, though," she'd reported to
Dr. Hoffman in satisfaction. Surprisingly, she'd said, the child
had shown the rooting reflex at the touch of the medicine dropper on its cheek—an almost unheard-of precocity in an infant
so small—and so, on her own initiative, Alice had perforated
the rubber cot of a dropper and allowed the baby to suckle,
which it did, though lapsing with fatigue after another cc.

Again, Dr. Hoffman shook his head in wonder. In his experience, girls generally fared better than boys, especially as
early independent feeders. He didn't like to argue with Alice,
who liked to see babies at the breast as early as possible, but
he was concerned that feeding the infant that way might

exhaust it. Though he'd gone ahead and asked Alice now about seeing to a wet nurse for the child, he thought he would resolve to go back to gavage if there were any problems. He'd rather see the baby get enough calories, at least, than wear itself out trying to nurse.

Though he had reminded Alice that babies sometimes came to them in unorthodox ways, he had to admit that he, too, had been surprised by this infant's method of arrival.

Alice had told him that she had just finished with the twelve o'clock showing and was turning back to her regular duties when she'd noticed a young man—presumably the child's father, though he never said as much—standing very still behind the rope partition. She'd been surprised, she said—the crowd had begun to move away through the exit, and she had imagined them all to be gone.

Sometimes women stayed behind, usually the ones who'd lost babies, Dr. Hoffman knew. He'd talked with plenty of them at Coney Island over the years. Poor, childless Rose Connell had been coming every day for eight years, all in the memory of the infant boy she'd lost over a decade before, a child she said had lived just three days, with no others ever to follow. They didn't charge her admission anymore, hadn't in years. She would sit in a corner and knit blankets for the babies, though Dr. Hoffman was loath to let her help in any other way. Her sadness, he thought, though not without regret or pity, made her too unreliable.

But *this* now, Alice said. This had been a young *man* lingering on behind.

Earlier that evening, Dr. Hoffman had returned to the hospital to find Alice waiting for him outside by the courtyard. He'd been to another unsuccessful dinner with the fair's scientific

board. Once again, the trustees had turned down his petition
to have his exhibit moved to the scientific quarter of the fair—
away from the freaks and dancing, he'd pleaded. *Please, gentlemen, consider your charge.*

Alice had been standing restlessly beside the fence when
Dr. Hoffman turned the corner by the Lido. A stork on the
other side of the fence, almost as tall as Alice and yet rail thin
beside her pale, doughy bulk, had looked out at Dr. Hoffman
as he'd approached through the dusk. He supposed Alice had
not seen him coming, because she startled when he spoke from
the shadows behind her.

"Does the stork have *many* interesting things to say?" he'd
asked her, teasing.

Alice had turned round. "He has nothing in his head but
feathers," she said, "but *I* have news for *you*."

And as Dr. Hoffman loosened his tie and mounted the steps
of the building, holding aside the door for Alice, she had told
him the story of the new baby's arrival.

She had been finishing with the noon showing, she'd said,
when she realized that one of the spectators had lingered behind in the gallery and was staring in at her. She had fixed him
with a questioning look. And then, she told Dr. Hoffman, he
had raised a *hatbox* toward her. A *hatbox!* And she had known
exactly what was inside it.

Motioning to the young man with her hand, she had hurried
around to the side door and admitted him, though she'd
stopped his progress with her foot when he started to move
deeper into the room. "We don't want germs in our nursery,"
she'd said.

"He looked terrible," she'd told Dr. Hoffman, as he took off
his jacket and handed it to her. "Dust all over his face and in
his hair—funny, wiry red hair. He had an odd face, like some-

one had taken a bite out of it, near his mouth. Looked like a bad tooth, to me. I knew what he had there with him, of course I did, and I thought how not to frighten him while still getting the child away from him. He was so short of breath, and his color wasn't good. 'Have you something with you, in your box?' I asked him at last, for he wouldn't say anything at first. And then he asked for you.

"I had to tell him you weren't here, of course," Alice went on, smoothing the folds in Dr. Hoffman's jacket. "'He'll be back this evening,' I told him, trying to soothe him. And finally, when he wouldn't say anything else, I asked him outright: 'Have you a baby in that box, sir!' He stared at me as though he couldn't imagine how I'd guessed it!"

Dr. Hoffman washed his hands while Alice stood behind him and talked, waving her big hands in the air, explaining. He moved the bar of soap up his arms and lathered heavily.

Alice hung Dr. Hoffman's jacket over a chair and picked up a towel from a cart. "And at last I had to say to him," she finished, " '*Will you give me your box, sir?*' "

Dr. Hoffman rinsed his arms. He cupped some water briefly in his palms and thought then of the statues with their open hands, their open mouths, in the fountains in the public gardens off the Alexanderplatz in Berlin, the wings of gray pigeons grazing the cheeks of the little stone children as the birds rose fluttering into the air. As a young child—his parents had moved their small family from Berlin to Paris when he was seven—he had been taken to the park with his nurse, and they had sat by the fountains on a bench. Every now and then, in a moment of shattering strangeness, he'd imagined that he'd seen one of the statues turn its cheek through a fan of water to look toward him. In that instant a thrilling hush would come over his body, as if he'd seen beyond death, beneath the porous and pocked skin of these stone children and into the quick, bright flame of their everlasting souls.

He let the water splash brightly, musically, into the enamel sink while he waited and listened. There wasn't another nurse as good as Alice, he thought, turning his attention toward her again, listening to her talk, but he supposed her manner might have intimidated the young man. He hoped not for good.

Alice gave him the clean towel when he turned around and held out his dripping hands to her.

"And then?" he asked. "So. You asked him for the box, and what did he do?"

When he finished drying his hands, Alice took the towel back from him and stood still for a moment, holding it. "Then he opened the box," she said. "He took off the lid and opened the box, and the baby was inside."

Dr. Hoffman rolled down his sleeves and buttoned his cuffs. "Alive."

"Alive." Alice took a breath and then turned away with an absent air, to put the damp towel into the hamper. "Yes, of course, it was alive." She turned back and looked at Dr. Hoffman. "And so I took the baby out and called for Nan."

"What did he do then? The father?"

Alice thought for a moment. "He just stood there, holding the empty box. 'It was alive when I left,' he said. 'I did my best with it. Sylvie'—I think that's the name he used, I suppose it's his wife—'and me and Mrs. Hermann'—that's the other person he mentioned—'we all done our best with it.' "

Dr. Hoffman frowned. "Didn't he understand the child was alive?"

"I don't know. He didn't really look at it. It was as if he didn't want to look at it." She paused. "I was so horrified. I suppose my reaction frightened him. Maybe he thought it was dead."

She turned away from Dr. Hoffman again and took a clean white gown from the stack on the table. "And then he just ran out the door, before I could say anything. He ran out the door holding the hatbox, and he never looked back."

Dr. Hoffman allowed Alice to help him into the gown.

"I called after him. 'Come back! You don't understand!' But he was gone." Alice turned an aggrieved face to Dr. Hoffman. "I'll be shocked if he comes back."

Dr. Hoffman frowned again. "He didn't tell you his name?"

Alice shook her head. "Only the wife's name, Sylvie. And that Mrs. Hermann he mentioned."

Dr. Hoffman began buttoning his gown. "Well, we could have the police inquire, I suppose," he said. "Though there must be hundreds of Hermanns in the city. And God knows how they would find a single woman named Sylvia."

"Sylvie," Alice corrected.

Hoffman glanced at her. "Yes. Of course."

"The odds are not very good, are they?" Alice looked pained.

Dr. Hoffman stopped. "No, not very good," he said. "But they never are, here, are they?"

"No," Alice said, and wiped her eyes. "No, I suppose they're not."

Looking in at the baby in his incubator now, Dr. Hoffman realized that Alice had probably been right. They were unlikely to see the child's parents again, even if they were to try to find them with the help of the police. He wanted to hope, though what *was* the point of saving them if no one wanted them? Alice had asked him this before, despairing over parents who paid regular visits for a while and then, over time, just gradually stopped coming. It was as if

the long weeks away from their babies were not a healing
time, not a cause for celebration, every day a miracle, but a
long, slow rupture, weeks when the child took on some iden-
tity that was not personal, not particular, but was, in a way,
more worldly. The child evolved, he thought, not into the
mother and father's child, *somebody's* flesh and blood, but
into a property of the world itself, a material like air or
sound. Yet each, he believed, possessed the heavy, individ-
ual heart of the orphan.

Sometimes he didn't even have an address and had no way
of finding the parents later, to try to persuade them to take
the children back. Once, back in Coney Island, he'd passed
a woman on the street near Surf Avenue in Sea Gate and
thought he recognized her as one of the mothers who'd abandoned her infant. He had stopped short, stared at her to be
sure, and then begun to cross the street to approach her, to tell
her that her boy, her infant Samuel, was now nearly eight
pounds, was in the orphanage, was well, and was waiting for
her! But she had seen him coming and had looked at him for a
moment with anguish and terror on her face. And then she
had picked up her skirts and run. He would not have run after
her, not for a minute. He was appalled that she feared him, as
a penitent later fears his confessor. It occurred to him that she
did not know whether the boy had lived or died. But still, for
Dr. Hoffman, who had held the infant, had coaxed it toward
term and then beyond, had seen it safely through the delicate
days of its too-soon time, the mother's response seemed inexplicable.

He had tried to tell Alice, though, that it didn't matter, didn't
matter whether anyone wanted them. They had a right to be in
the world, he thought, even if no one wanted them there except
the doctors and nurses who cared for them in their earliest

weeks, watching them drift inexorably toward death and then sometimes—surprisingly—rally. No, they had a right to be there, he thought, regardless of what the world would bring them, because they'd proved, already more than the average person, how much they wanted to be alive.

He surveyed the room around him. There they all were: Laura, 964 grams; tiny, black-haired Henry; gentle Pearl; Robert of the cleft palate; the one called C. K. by his devoted grandmother, a middle-aged woman whom Alice allowed to sit beside the incubator sometimes in the evenings, staring in at her grandson; the twins Adelaide and Agnes; John H. of the shriveled arm; John B., already a handsome boy, unusual in these infants who were so often ugly; Bernice, who was certain to be blind; little dark-skinned Helen; Leonore, whose convulsions seemed to be falling in number now at last, thank God. He knew them all, knew how their temperatures had risen and fallen, knew how much milk they took, how much oxygen, how much protein. He'd seen their blood, the little streams of it wicking away like blue ink under their thin skin. He saw personalities in them already, the ones who were patient and dazzled by the bright lights, the ones who roughed up their faces and mewled their fury at the world, the ones who turned and rooted at the pad of his thumb when he held it to their mouths, the ones who lay still, very still, as if inside a shell.

Now the lights of the room had been dimmed. The white rocking chairs were empty, still. The glass doors of the incubators shone with a wet black gleam, the swaddled infants within motionless as sarcophagi. The wet nurses, having offered a final feeding until the next at two in the morning, had retired with their own pink-cheeked infants and their heavy breasts to the apartment set aside for them in one of the side wings of the building.

Upon arriving in Chicago earlier that month, Dr. Hoffman had been disturbed to discover, despite his requesting otherwise, that the room for the twelve wet nurses had been constructed simply as one long, grim dormitory. He had wanted to offer his wet nurses the privacy of rooming with only one other mother—a luxury he supposed would be a welcome novelty for many of them. He had wanted flowers in their rooms, a pretty view perhaps, pictures on the walls. He had wanted some measure of comfort afforded them, these women who allowed themselves to be pumped like cows for their milk, their breasts blue and straining at the rubber cups, these women who would cheerfully suckle a lamb, a wolf, the whole world, he thought. He handled the glass tubes of their breast milk, held the chilled vials in his hand and saw the rich cream collect at the top, each time with a sense of pleasure at the natural order of things, a respect for the perfect pattern of provision that lay beneath the untidy business people made of bearing children.

He had asked specifically for at least six separate chambers, even if very small, and a window for each room, and had been furious when he inspected the building and found instead the stark dormitory. Still, the women didn't seem to mind. They formed a queer, temporary sisterhood, he observed, each seated in a rocker, chatting away with her neighbor, her shirtwaist untied, a breast held loosely in her hand and extended toward a tiny mouth. They lost all sense of embarrassment at his presence among them and allowed him inspection of their breasts and mammilla. Those with small but protuberant nipples, he found, were the most satisfactory for starting an infant being weaned from gavage.

His own apartment was grander than he found necessary, even embarrassingly so. He suspected that Dr. Ludwig, who had promised to report on the construction to Dr. Hoffman, had discovered the error in the quarters for the wet nurses and had tried belatedly to compensate for Dr. Hoffman's disappointment by ordering a more lavish apartment for Dr. Hoffman himself, including loaning him his own cook and a chauffeur for the duration of the exposition. Still, Dr. Hoffman had been grateful for Dr. Ludwig's solicitousness and especially for the small walled garden he'd seen added to Dr. Hoffman's private wing.

At night, after making his final rounds, Dr. Hoffman would sit sometimes at the wrought iron table and chair on the flagstones of the garden and have a glass of wine before retiring. Dr. Ludwig, with his customary fastidiousness, had seen to everything, Dr. Hoffman thought with gratitude, including four enormous African pots bearing trained bougainvilleas in full bloom which had been set out on the little terrace. Dr. Ludwig would know his friend Leo would appreciate that. Two mimosa trees on the far side of the garden wall draped their delicate greenery over his table, casting a pretty, rippling shadow across the flagstones at night. He'd noticed, too, that Dr. Ludwig had asked that a small statue of Saint Nicholas, patron saint of children, be installed in a shallow alcove of the wall. The statue's expression was bland, its palms turned outward as if it were apologizing for the limits of its responsibility. All this Dr. Hoffman cast his eyes over as he sat in the garden in the evenings, waiting for the day's exertions to drain away from him and leave him restful enough for sleep.

Sitting in this private garden at the end of his day, he could hear the fair crowds on the other side of the wall making their way from one amusement to the next as night wore on toward morning, the sky changing gradually from a dusty black to a deep, cerulean blue and finally to fluid bars of pink and yellow crossed with pale striations of clouds as the sun rose again. At night, while the moon climbed overhead and the stars came out, Dr. Hoffman could hear shrieks and laughter, the ominous sounds of arguments that drained away, as often as not, into a drunken tenderness. The surging, gay sounds of the piano or saxophone or drums, as doors swung open and closed all along the avenues of the Streets of Paris, seemed far away as he sat and reviewed the day's events in his head. Sometimes he was late enough to catch the exposition's final show of the evening, the Northern Lights display, in the pale dome of sky overhead. He would take off his shoes at the door and walk in his black socks across the cool stones. Seated at his table, he could look down into his glass of burgundy to see faint explosions of reflected color ripple across the surface of his wine.

Now he backed away from the incubator holding the new infant and sat down in one of the rockers. He removed his glasses. Alice and four other nurses, including a young woman whose name he could never remember, sat at their station at the far end of the room under a low lamp, making notes in the infants' charts. Nan Silverman, who'd come with him from Coney Island, circulated quietly like an angel in her starched white uniform among the incubators, adjusting coverings, checking temperatures. The room was quiet.

Physicians were often surprised, after regular hospital nurseries, by the silence of the premature babies. The heavy stillness made doctors nervous, though Dr. Hoffman himself had learned to tell by sight, as had his nurses, whether the silence was simply the sweet peacefulness of sleep or the unnatural arrest of the heart and lungs. Alice, who had a kind of sixth sense for it, Dr. Hoffman thought, had been known to cross the room suddenly to revive at a single touch of her finger an infant who had lapsed. He explained to his colleagues—though some would not call themselves his peers, he knew, seeing his work in the public sphere as coarse and undignified—that protest or desire requires energy to make itself known; he believed his infants sensible to the cost to themselves of vocal grief.

Still, it unnerved him sometimes, too, the relative noiselessness of the nursery, especially in the evening. It was Alice's notion to try to accustom the babies to the regular rhythms of day and night, to dim the lights gradually as night fell, and to raise them gently again at sunrise. Yet Dr. Hoffman could never rid himself of the feeling that the babies were not sleeping, not really. They were waiting, he felt. And not for something general and unimagined, some disturbance in the street outside or even in the heavens themselves. They were waiting for him. He was dismayed at the self-interested quality of this sensation on his part, though he was quick to ascribe the tendency to what Dr. Ludwig laughingly called his "lonely vigil on the circus frontier of premature medicine."

Still, sitting there now in the quiet nursery, gazing around him at this public spectacle of human frailty and bravery, of life and death, at this place that he had created not as a means of self-aggrandizement but as a necessary shrine to medical investigation—in the absence, he reminded himself, *of any other means of support*—he could not rid himself of the feeling that these tiny babies were, though without the learned tools of language, asking him something with the one common tongue of their understanding: their hearts. But what was it, he thought, rubbing his eyes. What did they want from him?

• • •

With some embarrassment, he realized he had fallen asleep. He opened his eyes, saw Alice and another nurse still bent over their table, the lead from their pencils scratching faintly across the paper. Dr. Hoffman shifted carefully in his chair, a disguised stretch, and raised his gaze to the incubator before him.

And then, his own eyes struggling through the confusing grid of shadowy reflections cast over the dark glass—slashes of black and white, the tiny yellow orb of the distant lamp under which Alice worked at the far side of the room, the endless repeating pattern of the other silvery incubators with their motionless occupants—he saw the child's eyes regarding him.

He put on his glasses, hooked them over his ears, leaned forward. A transparent image of his own face flared in the glass, the eyes searching. But yes, he had been right. The infant was awake, lying on its side, and staring at him. Its eyes were a grave and beautiful blue, he saw, the dark color of the ocean before a storm. But the face—once more he was struck by how ancient the face of the premature baby was, like something uncovered beneath a rock by the side of the sea to be consulted about the birth of the planet. The prematures had none of the innocence and happiness that fat and flesh can confer to the face.

Dr. Hoffman craned over in the rocking chair, put his hand slowly to the glass. The child didn't blink, and for a second Dr. Hoffman's adrenaline rose and he was seized with fear. But then he saw the baby's hand, still curled near its cheek, spasm involuntarily. A little shudder ran over its jaw. Dr. Hoffman stood and opened the door of the incubator. Reaching in, he extended his fingers and placed the full length of his palm over the infant's body, his fingertips resting on the uneven seam of the child's head, his middle finger seeking the soft, throbbing fontanel at the top of the child's skull. The baby's eyelids closed once and then opened again, though it failed to follow the shifting plane of Dr. Hoffman's face, staring now instead into his shirtfront, the pearl buttons glinting against the starched white cotton. The little body under his hand shifted slightly, a relaxing, settling, spreading movement, as if it were trying to fill Dr. Hoffman's hand, to bring all parts of itself into contact with Dr. Hoffman's palm.

Dr. Hoffman didn't often hold the babies. He didn't have time. That's what Alice and the other nurses were for; and Alice had always stressed the importance of this, the surmounting need these babies had for human contact. He saw the value of it, yet it was not a function he often fulfilled. Sometimes, when he wanted certain kinds of information from a baby, the sort he could get only by looking at it, he would carry one for a while, pacing around the nursery, not exactly looking at the baby but all the while coming to know it. His hands and body registered the infant's strength and reflexes, its aspect of vigor or apathy. He could feel a fever or chill with his hands, could feel gastrointestinal difficulty and pain, could discern retractions in the ribs when a baby struggled to breathe. He could predict an apneic attack and forestall it with minute doses of carbon dioxide. He prescribed prophylactic vitamins D and K, intramuscular doses of crude liver extract, ferrous salts for anemia, ampoules of alpha lobeline for asphyxia neonatorum. His armamentarium was fully stocked. Yet the wave of information that washed over him when he held a child was sometimes so thick, so dense with signals and suggestions and implications, that he felt giddy from it, like a medium in the grip of a spirit's hand. Could he predict, he thought, the whole lifetime of the child in his arms? It almost seemed to him that he could, and sometimes he had to close his eyes

against a train of random, unbidden images leaping up before
him—falls from trees and races across the running spaces of
fields, a finger following the letters on a page, two heels flexing
against the deck of a ship, arms bearing loads of wash, or a
chicken gripped by the neck in two strong hands. He saw body
parts, magically grown from the miniature limbs he saw every
day into full, adult sizes—arms wreathed with coarse black
hair, legs carved with muscle. Yet always their faces—the
faces of the adults they would become—remained out of reach
for him.

He had gentle hands, as if his fingertips themselves were
aware of the fragile capillaries of these children and how easily
they bruised. Alice had told him he had the hands of her
grandfather, a gentle man who had handled pet canaries all his
life. Nurses said of Dr. Hoffman that his presence had an instantly calming effect on agitated babies. He was aware of this
capacity in himself and tried to use it when he had the time,
but he did not consider it magical, or even a gift, only the
transmission from himself to these babies of some comforting
authority, the authority any adult has, he imagined, for any
child. Sometimes—though only very rarely, for it made him
uncomfortable—he wondered why he did not feel *more* emotional attachment to his charges. His nurses cried when babies
died, but he did not. He thought that perhaps he could not afford to. He was too busy.

So he was surprised now, his hand covering this newcomer's
tiny body, at the sudden pricking at the corners of his eyes.
Beneath his palm he felt the laboring of the infant's lungs, the
racing accelerations of the child's heart, the invisible dispersal
of oxygen throughout the organs, the exploding production of
red blood cells. The little eyes, naked as a statue's, stared
ahead as if encountering the future on a stained glass window,

a moving picture of possibilities. Slowly, Dr. Hoffman leaned over to bring his face within the infant's view. And as he met its eyes, a strange curiosity rose up in his own heart. *What is it that you know?*

A kind of chill ran over him, a humility he hadn't experienced in a long, long time, not since his earliest days in medical school, his first harrowing months in residency. Since beginning his own hospital, he had been simply overwhelmed—and made bold, perhaps, he thought now—by how much he learned every day, with each infant, with every observation, every death, every survival. There almost hadn't been time to be humble, a truth that struck him now with a grim irony.

The infant closed its eyes.

And then, with a surprising fervor, Dr. Hoffman made a sudden wish on behalf of this child, on behalf of himself.

Don't die on me, he wished then. *You're not the smallest baby I've ever seen. You're just . . .*

But it took him a moment to realize what it was, what distinguished this child from any of the others who had come under his care over the years. He understood, at last, the quality that made him feel suddenly so uncertain in its presence.

In every other case, even when the mothers were young, too young to be mothers themselves, or when they were poor, or unintelligent, or certain their babies would die—in every single other case, he'd had one thing to start with, the thing that gave him entry to the child, its past, present, and future.

But he did not even know this baby's name. He did not know whether it had ever been given a name. He put his fingers to the glass of the incubator.

For the time being, he thought, *you're just the hatbox baby.*

FOUR

Late that evening, after checking the babies' charts, Dr. Hoffman stepped out of the nursery and into the hall. Pausing there to take off his glasses and fold them up into his pocket, he registered once again the impermanence of the space around him. In the spaces open to the public or set aside, as in the case of Dr. Hoffman's own apartment, for living quarters, the fair buildings appeared entirely finished. But they were really more like stage sets; in this hallway, for instance, only the rudest materials had been used. The light fixtures were few and without ornament, the floor was bare, the walls were roughly plastered and unpainted. The contrast between the two areas—one bright and inhabited, carefully detailed, and the other with its crude, almost abandoned quality —produced in Dr. Hoffman a feeling of self-consciousness. When he entered the nursery, or even his own rooms, it was like stepping onto a temporary stage, a place that might easily vanish when he wasn't there. He put his palm lightly, experimentally, against the wall beside him and was struck by the notion that it might move under his hand, sliding back to reveal yet another hallway, an endless series of them perhaps, each as unfinished and impermanent as this one. He took his hand away and brushed a film of dust from his palm.

Though he had nodded off in the chair in the nursery, he found himself alert now, in the agitated way of one who has slept just a few moments and has then been awakened suddenly. He wasn't sleepy. He would, he decided, walk for a short while before retiring. He let himself out of the building and stood on the flight of steps before the front door, watching the storks. For all their ugliness, he agreed with Alice's observation that the creatures had a patient, parental quality, like people who find themselves surprised by a new baby late in life. As Dr. Hoffman bent and lit a match for his pipe—his nightly indulgence—one of the tall birds stepped away from the shadows by the railing and waded slowly into the little lagoon sunk into the center of the imprisoned garden. The lights of the fair were still blazing; rings of colored light circled the streetlamps, bright blue and yellow and red and violet, like the spectrum flame of a gas torch. Dr. Hoffman supposed that the birds would retire at last when the lights were finally turned off and the streets were quiet. He watched as the stork dropped its long neck until its bill met the water and then froze there to drink, motionless as a figure in a frieze. Whose idea had *this* been, bringing these poor birds here? Each day must feel never-ending.

Dr. Hoffman pulled his watch from his pocket and checked the time. It was just past midnight. He would walk for only a few minutes, he promised himself, and then go to bed. Recently, Dr. Ludwig had sent over a young medical resident, Dr. Sandor, from his staff at Sarah Morris to assist Dr. Hoffman at night; this meant that for the first time in what felt like his lifetime,

Dr. Hoffman was able to sleep all night long if he wished. Oddly, though, he'd found himself almost incapable of doing this. He often woke two or three times during the night, sometimes so sufficiently that he had to get up and sit in his garden for a while or turn on the light by his bed and read. He kept Marcus Aurelius's *Meditations* on his nightstand; he found the force of will behind the youthful Roman emperor's prescriptions comforting: "Dig within," he read at night lying in bed, the book propped open on his knees. "There lies the wellspring of good: ever dig, and it will ever flow."

Occasionally he would return to the nursery in the middle of the night to go over the infants' charts or check on a baby he was particularly worried about, but Dr. Ludwig had heard about this and told him he'd take back the young resident if Dr. Hoffman didn't stay in bed.

"You're forty years old, Dr. Hoffman," Dr. Ludwig had chided his friend. "Come on, Leo," he'd continued, dropping the customary title of *Dr.* to signal both his fondness and his personal concern in this matter. "You've earned a good night's sleep, for God's sake."

Consequently, Dr. Hoffman was trying to develop the semblance of a normal schedule, retiring around midnight and sleeping until six or so.

He'd discovered that he much preferred the fair at night. Some of it was the heat; it was staggeringly hot already this summer, and the fair had just opened. He couldn't imagine how hot it might be in July and August. At least at night when the sun went down there was some relief from the thick air. But by midnight the crowds had thinned out, and he could walk along the street at his own characteristically brisk pace, without pausing for people ahead of him. Tonight he stopped to relight his pipe and then proceeded.

He had to give the architects and planners of the fair credit; glancing around at the gabled storefronts and neat buildings, he realized that the Streets of Paris, where tourists were supposed to imagine themselves in Europe, looked reasonably authentic. If the crowds had been less American in appearance, anyone might have been fooled into thinking he was truly on the Continent.

Yet, as he looked more closely, he seemed to sense rather than actually see a small, almost negligible fault: the scale was not quite right. The buildings were too small; the areas between the doors and the windows too narrow, the rooflines too shallow. And now he noticed that the people on the street seemed, by comparison, a little too large, either fatter or taller than they should be, their features more pronounced. The error was not sufficient to make this disparity vulgar or really even noticeable if you weren't paying attention. But Dr. Hoffman noticed it now, this jarring of perspective. Trying to account for it was impossible, though, like trying to account for the unexplainable elements of a dream in which the curious is commonplace and the dreamer's incredulity is a sign of his own madness.

He had to stop now on the sidewalk and step aside politely as a trio of young women sashayed toward him under the milky glow of the streetlights, their arms around one another's waists. They were singing. The tallest of the three, nearest Dr. Hoffman, had a high white forehead, her heavy dark hair pinned in a loose, wide roll at the nape of her neck. Her red dress fitted closely around the waist, low at the bodice in a crossed V that displayed the tops of her breasts, the bluish gorge of her clavicle and throat. Her cheeks were flushed a dark red; her nostrils flared. She sang with her eyes closed and her head

thrown back, her companions singing along as well and laughing, tripping over one another's feet.

Dr. Hoffman stepped close to the wall. As they passed him,
the tall girl in red swayed toward his shirtfront. She opened her
eyes suddenly and paused for a beat, a mocking expression on
her face. And then they were past, a six-legged creature weaving away under the streetlights. Young men hopped down off
the curb to get out of their way, looked back over their shoulders, and whistled.

Dr. Hoffman glanced down at his pipe. Had it gone out? The
passing of the three girls could only have taken a minute, and
yet he felt aged by the encounter. The movements of another
passerby, a glass descending slowly in glittering revolutions
from a café tabletop to the pavement, a voice hurtling down the
street—all these occurred only in his peripheral attention,
distant signals from another time and place. Then a boy, running with wide strides like a hurdler, crossed Dr. Hoffman's
path in pursuit of a handful of coins flung from somewhere, the
coins turning in the heavy night air and then beginning their
descent, the boy, his hands outstretched, determined to catch
them before they reached the ground and were lost under the
feet of pedestrians. Three waiters, their arms folded over their
white shirts—one with his foot resting on the low stone wall of
the café's terrace—were laughing at the boy.

Dr. Hoffman was unused to the bustle of the streets. The
nursery was so quiet that the confusing activity of the outside
world often left him in a daze. But there was something else
that needed to be said, he thought, something else about how
he saw all this—but what would he call it? All this *what?*
What was it? He struggled to be certain. It was only, he
thought, only that sometimes it all seemed—so unimportant.

Is that what he believed? That it was—even his own
endeavor—unimportant? Sometimes, perhaps because his responsibilities felt so great, or because the odds were so poor, or
because his patients were so helpless and so innocent, he felt
that he had become something he had never intended to become when he set out to be a doctor. He never took any money
for the babies' care. But he could tell, he had learned to tell,
those who would die anyway and those who would be damaged
despite his efforts. Sometimes he felt he stood pointlessly between the fragile world of living things and some great, res-
olute force that was slowly trying to crush him against the wall
of its own intractable conviction.

He shook his head. What good were such thoughts? He
reached slowly to tap the bowl of his pipe against the wall. A
meager shower of faint red sparks fell silently toward the pavement, extinguishing itself on its descent. *Those girls,* he thought,
that tall girl in red . . . but he was not accustomed to thinking
of women. He had no time for women other than the generous
mothers who fed all his babies. When he thought about women
at all, it was to promise himself that one day, when the Coney
Island hospital was running exactly as he liked, when he wasn't
traveling so much—then he'd look for a wife. He'd had one
love affair while in medical school in Paris; he had felt grateful
beyond expression to the generous girl, a native Berliner, like
himself, who had allowed him to discover her body. But that
had been, oh, almost twenty years ago.

Could he even remember her name?

Gretel, he thought suddenly in relief. *Her name was Gretel.*

He began to walk again, sucking on his pipe, looking down
at the pavement. He saw only the Indians' beaded moccasins
as the men passed him, six or seven of them. The tassels on
their leather chaps were stained and dirty, but the beads on

their slippers—red and white and yellow—shone up from the pavement like fool's gold.

Three couples, the women with their arms linked through the elbows of their men, strolled down the sidewalk ahead of him. The women's heels sounded a fusillade of small, tight reports. A pool of dark shadows thrown by their skirts advanced ahead of them. Dr. Hoffman slowed down briefly before stepping off the curb to pass them, and he heard the soft tones of their conversation, their light, amiable laughter.

He was tired, that was all; Dr. Ludwig had said he looked tired, and Dr. Hoffman supposed it was true. The previous afternoon, when he had walked over to the Hall of Science to look longingly at the exhibit space there, he had seen himself reflected in the mirrors in the main gallery; across the huge central hall he had stopped, momentarily perplexed. Was that *him?* Stooped and slow-moving, like an old man? So, yes, he was tired. There had been problems at the Coney Island hospital—the young doctor he'd hired to maintain things there had offended two of his oldest nurses. One baby there had died unexpectedly following a seizure. There were all these babies here to worry about. And now this new baby . . . the hatbox baby.

But it wasn't even all that, though any of it might have been enough, he saw, to make a man feel tired. This discomfort, this loneliness—really, if he was honest with himself, they had always been there. He could subdue them by work, the honorableness of his work, the gravity of his responsibility. But they were there, he knew with regret—these tendencies. He did not like to think of himself as a man who was flawed in this way, for it did not seem to him that he could do anything about it. Nothing he had ever done—not even saving lives—had changed this essential quality of his nature, this anxiety.

The sidewalk in front of him had become crowded. Just up the street, the doors of the Lido had opened, and people who'd been to see the fan dancer's last show of the night stepped out under the streetlights, from darkness into the artificial brightness of the street, blinking and casting about as if they expected to be met or as if they hoped to see someone they knew.

Dr. Hoffman slowed his pace, impeded by the crowd now moving sluggishly toward him.

People spilled out into the street, a close mass of bodies under the white haze of the streetlights, cyclones of tiny insects gathering overhead. Here and there in the crowd, men stopped up short to hunch their shoulders and cup their hands to light a cigarette. Women in flowered dresses waited beside them; they gazed off into some indeterminate distance, fanning clouds of scent from their hair and their moist necks, their skirts swaying. Dr. Hoffman began to step out into the street to get away from the closeness of the crowd, but there were just as many people there, too, filling the street practically from curb to curb. All these people—just to see a woman dance with ostrich feathers? He began to edge his way through the flow of pedestrians coming toward him in a wave; the noise of them was deafening. Why were they being so *loud?* He found himself cursing the fan dancer for spoiling his walk.

Then a jostling movement on the far side of the crowd buoyed up to the surface; a few people turned their heads, stepped back. Dr. Hoffman nearly collided with a slender woman in a white dress. How had she managed to stay so clean, he wondered; the skirt of her dress was folded into hundreds of complicated little pleats, her hair cropped daringly short, like a boy's. She leaned toward him, solicitous, as if she recognized him and would offer condolence. He stopped, surprised.

"Hey! Watch it!" A young man shouldering past Dr. Hoffman, with jug ears and a loose white shirt rolled past the elbows, turned around, waiting for a fight. He put up his hands and shoved a tall fellow, thin as a snake, who had jostled into the jug-eared boy as the crowd shifted.

Dr. Hoffman's anger mounted. Foolishness. They'd only start trouble.

But the thin man stumbled again, pushed forward by those behind him; he stepped on the heel of the jug-eared boy's companion, a plump, black-haired girl scarcely more than a child, with a thickly painted mouth and a sullen expression. She cried out, turning around and scowling at Dr. Hoffman as if he had been responsible. "Why don'tcha—"

"Yeah," the jug-eared boy said, giving the thin man a second shove, angry. "Who do—"

"Sorry!" The fellow glanced behind him. "It's not *my* fault."

The crowd gathering around them had achieved the thickness of fog; why didn't people just move along? Dr. Hoffman tried to turn around, to go back the way he had come. He would go home, back to his walled garden. His walk had been spoiled. Sweat had broken out along his brow. He mopped at his face. Then the crowd shifted again, a live mass like a single creature, its perimeters bulging. Dr. Hoffman looked up; the streetlights overhead buzzed as if a timer had been started, and under their deafening noise, all other sounds faded away into silence. Dr. Hoffman turned slowly; patrons at the café across the street were standing up, the men with their napkins in their hands. One woman, her hand to her mouth, reached up desperately for her companion's sleeve and hung on. Where had this crowd come from? How had this happened?

And then the silence broke. Or rather Dr. Hoffman himself

seemed to emerge from underwater into the night air laced with sharp voices, a babble of orders and entreaties. A ripple of fear spread through the crowd, brushed past Dr. Hoffman, and left him speechless. People around him stumbled, caught at one another. Dr. Hoffman saw hands flashing, felt his own pulse begin to race as voices were raised around him. A man, two women, fell in the street near him, trampled underfoot as the crowd shifted away from some fierce center; Dr. Hoffman heard a single cry, a man's voice tempered to a high pitch in fear. "Oh God. Oh God."

But Dr. Hoffman could see nothing. He bent over instinctively to offer his arm to one of the women who had fallen and was crying; he had to yank her arm to pull her up quickly, out from under the trampling feet of the crowd. He felt in his own shoulder the pain he had probably caused her. He had to stagger to keep his own balance against the force of people now fleeing in every direction, women screaming, men shouting. A stench of alcohol and sweat and perfume and spoiling food met Dr. Hoffman's nostrils as he came painfully to his knees in the street, knocked down by the crowd. He was surprised; he couldn't remember the last time he'd been on his hands and knees—it must have been in childhood. And then a scream, loosened from a man's throat, rose up over the shouting and confusion.

"He's got a knife!" someone shouted.

Dr. Hoffman struggled to his feet, looked around wildly. Faces rushed past him, white and distorted.

A voice rang out, raw with desperation. "This man needs a doctor! Somebody get a doctor!"

Dr. Hoffman found his voice. "Here," he called. "Here. I am a doctor." The people nearest him turned and stared as if in disbelief. It was the accent, the trace of eastern Europe that clung to his consonants. People distrusted accents; but they parted to let him through.

A man lay on the street. Dr. Hoffman shouldered through the crowd and dropped to his knees at the man's side. The wound in the man's stomach was deep and long and fatal, a messy knife wound beginning just beneath the ribs and angling upward in a practiced thrust toward the heart and lungs. He lay on his back, one knee bent, his arms fallen open loosely on either side of him in a gesture of abandon. Dr. Hoffman recognized the position. It was the same posture premature infants fell into when laid upon their backs. With such poor muscle tone, there was nothing to keep the limbs flexed. They fell open as if they lacked joints.

Dark blood streamed from the man's nostrils and mouth, pooled into his ears and hair—a wiry, brittle red hair, unusual in texture and color. Dr. Hoffman leaned over and put two fingers to the slender neck of the man—a boy, really, for he seemed to be young now, as Dr. Hoffman drew near, and growing younger every moment as his heart slowed, as his blood ebbed from him and lay over the stones. Dr. Hoffman felt the pulse throb heavily, its painful decelerations. He heard the uneven rasp of the boy's breath, the sound of a far-off sawing, deep in a forest. There wasn't anything anyone could do.

"It's bad?" Another man, kneeling beside Dr. Hoffman at the injured boy's head, spoke. He was white-faced; his lips trembled. He held a blue handkerchief in his hand, had touched it to the wounded boy's lips. Now it was stained with blood.

Dr. Hoffman glanced at him. "He is your friend?"

But the older man shook his head and then covered his face with his hands. "No," he said. "I don't even know him."

Dr. Hoffman touched the boy's chest gently. "What happened?"

The man took his hands away, wiped his sleeve across his face. "Jesus," he said fiercely. "There were so many people all of a sudden, everybody shoving. I don't know. It was like—he was in the way."

The strangeness of this remark did not appear to strike the man, and Dr. Hoffman could not tell exactly what he had meant—whether the victim himself had blocked this man's view or, worse, the dying boy had been, as this man now said, simply *in the way*, a body taking up the wrong space, a body that should not have been there.

Dr. Hoffman looked down. The injured boy's head and neck and chest convulsed, his legs jerked spasmodically. One eye flashed open, rolled. "Steady," Dr. Hoffman said now, leaning close. "Rest. Shhh." He hushed him, the dying boy, as he hushed the babies. And he thought of Deveaux, the doctor he had most admired throughout the years of his training. "Look at the *eyes*, my young friends. 'The lamp of the body is the eye.'" And Deveaux would lift a patient's eyelid, direct a beam into the pupil, which contracted, cringing, against the glare of inspection. "From the Bible, in *case* you don't already know," Deveaux would say, with his characteristically odd inflections. "Matthew. Chapter *six*, verse *twenty*-two."

The boy's hands came up briefly in the air, the parallel palms of the minister waiting, waiting, waiting for the congregants to come to their knees, to begin to pray.

Dr. Hoffman ripped open the boy's shirt. The man beside him wretched, turned his head away. Dr. Hoffman was faintly aware, as he bent over the boy's body and probed the wound, of the sound of people crying, two or three voices muffled in shirtfronts, behind hands.

He looked down into the face of the boy beneath him. What on earth could this boy have done to deserve this? How

slender he was, wrists like a girl and a delicate neck. He noted
the boy's chin: the evidence of a poor surgeon or poor care or
both, the triangle of collapsed flesh over the jawline where a frag-
ment of bone had been sacrificed to the operation. The poor
always suffer so from fools and incompetent surgeons, he
thought. "Get an ambulance, please," he said shortly, without
looking up, to the man shaking and kneeling beside him.

The man scrambled to his feet; the crowd was already calling for an ambulance. Not that there was anything to be done,
Dr. Hoffman thought.

He had been *in the way*, the man had said. In the way of
what? Or who? Was there a chain of worthiness, so that one
soul truly might be more valuable than the next? As deaths
went, Dr. Hoffman thought, there were certainly worse than
this, deaths more drawn out and excruciating, deaths that
ridiculed a dignified man, deaths that humiliated the modest,
deaths that suffocated and terrified.

But this—he touched the boy's forehead lightly with his
thumb—this death would be more like a dream.

Dr. Hoffman pulled at his collar. He was sweating heavily;
drops ran down his nose. It was preposterous: how could standing too close, or even shoving—if this boy were guilty of
either—have earned him this, this trickling away on the street,
the contents of his heart evaporating into the close, still air of
the night. What had happened here? People were leaving the
theater on a summer night, heading for home or a last drink—
it was hot, they were all a little too close together, people were
tired. And one of them took a knife and drove it up into the
heart of the man beside him. Was that *it?*

Dr. Hoffman was used to death, he told himself. But not murder. He bowed his head over the boy, put up the back of his
hand to stanch the river of sweat running down his temples.

When he looked up, he saw that a tight circle of onlookers had closed in around him. They stared down at him, their lips closed, their faces grave. The crowns of their heads, shining under the streetlights, were valiant and bright, but dark hollows collected beneath their eyes. Dr. Hoffman swallowed, aware suddenly of a most fundamental thirst.

"Does anyone know this man?" He spoke quietly, searching the faces bent over him. One or two people stepped back, as if to avoid his eyes. A few shook their heads slowly. No one answered, and Dr. Hoffman looked away from them.

Carefully, he folded the boy's torn shirt over the wound. He would not survive this, Dr. Hoffman knew. He would be fortunate if he lived only another few minutes.

He took the boy's hand, raised it in his own, wrapped his fingers around the cooling palm. It was what he knew to do for the dying, what he did with the babies. He lifted their hands, fit his big thumb into the grip of their tiny palms, leaned over them. "Hold on," he said to them. "Hold on." And sometimes they did.

When he sensed a movement in the crowd, he glanced up. He thought it might be the man he had sent off, returning with a stretcher and some extra hands. But as he looked at the ring of people around him, it broke open, and a woman, clad in only a silk kimono, her feet in a pair of fur-trimmed mules, broke through the crowd and stood staring down at him, a horrified expression on her face.

"My God," she said, and folded her arms. It was a funny gesture; at first Dr. Hoffman thought she meant to be disapproving. Then he realized she was trying to prevent herself from shaking. The crowd moved back, almost deferentially.

"What happened?" she said. She did not look at Dr. Hoffman but stared down at the boy.

She was beautiful, but in a way that surprised Dr. Hoffman. She had a wide mouth like a bowstring drawn back. She seemed—she seemed to fit her skin perfectly. That was it. Her hair, a thick, rich brown the color of maple syrup, was damp at the ends. Her eyes were black.

"I didn't see it," he said. "Do you know him?"

She shook her head.

"He was at your show, Miss Day," a small voice in the crowd said quietly. "He sat beside me."

The woman glanced over her shoulder into the crowd as if to determine who had spoken, but the information appeared not to interest her much. "Someone's gone to get a doctor?" she said, turning back and speaking to Dr. Hoffman.

"I am a doctor."

She met his eyes, stared at him. "Oh . . ."

Her hair flew out around her head in an odd nimbus, the streetlamp framing her in a silvery glare, exposing the fullness of her figure through the thin robe. And then he realized who she was, who she must be: the fan dancer.

He had not ever expected to meet her. That he had found his nursery located next to the Lido, where she held her show, dancing naked behind two big ostrich-feather fans, had infuriated him, as it always did to have his hospital placed in the same category as cheap entertainments like that. When he had first begun his work with premature infants, such fairs, especially those in Europe, were more serious. He had felt flattered— appropriately, he thought—by the invitations, and he hadn't minded the trouble of the temporary installments. In fact, he had enjoyed the sense he had of being both a pioneer and a teacher. That the public was willing to pay to see the babies—that was well and good, as there weren't funds coming from anywhere else. With his public shows, he had amassed more equipment, saved more premature babies, than any other doctor.

But that the organizers of this fair—the Century of *Progress,* no less, he thought bitterly—imagined that he and a fan dancer had something in common. It baffled and outraged him.

He stared back at her. She was older than he might have expected, he saw; this startled him, too. She fell back a bit under his inspection. And then he shrugged, inclined his head to the side very slightly, made a frowning gesture with his mouth to imply their complicity—they both understood that this man would die. He saw her catch his meaning and felt obscurely pleased by this. Behind her, the crowd shrank away. They, too, understood.

But the fan dancer surprised him then by kneeling suddenly on the bloody pavement beside him and taking the man's head between her palms, putting her mouth close to his ear. He could not catch her words, only the low, comforting murmur of her voice. He was reminded of Alice, how she held the babies they knew were dying, how she spoke to them, taking them out on the sound of her voice, speaking of ordinary things.

Her hair fell over the young man's bloodied lips.

And then Dr. Hoffman, still holding the boy's hand, felt the boy's fingers fly open, a gesture of astonishment, as if the hands needed to be ready to catch hold of a rising scaffold and climb, or receive a shower of light, or find with their fingertips the familiar face of someone this boy knew. For he would be blind now, blinded by the light, and going too quickly, in any case, to see.

"Steady," Dr. Hoffman said low, and he meant it now not as a stay, but as instruction for a voyager, a sailor who must hold the tiller in a wild sea. "Steady."

When he took his eyes at last from the young man's face, the face settling in an instant into a cold permanence, he looked up, expecting to meet the fan dancer's eyes. What was her name? He could not remember her name. She was the best-known woman in Chicago that summer. *What was her name?*

But she did not look at him again. She sat back on her heels, her face impassive. Then, gathering her filthy, ruined robe close around her throat, she stood up. She looked down at the boy for a moment. And then she turned and walked away, the crowd parting ahead of her.

As she neared the door of the Lido, a man stepped up to her, an autograph book and a pen held in his hand. "Autograph, Miss Day?" he said, holding out the pen.

Dr. Hoffman saw her look at the man; her face was astonishingly void of expression. And then she took the pen from his hand, and the book, and bent over and wrote something on the page. *Could the man not see that she was covered in blood?* But she wrote carefully, as if she'd never learned to write her name quickly and each time had to fashion the letters in unfamiliar curving loops and curlicues. When she had finished, she handed the book back to the man, who grinned. "Thanks!"

She did not smile back. She didn't even look at him. And in a minute she had disappeared inside.

At that moment, the man Dr. Hoffman had sent off before returned with two policemen and a squad car. An ambulance trailed behind, filling the street with a clanging of bells. The crowd quieted; it was nearly over now. Dr. Hoffman spoke briefly to the first policeman, a man with a thick black mustache, his shirt straining over his belly. "Poor kid," the policeman said, looking down at the boy while his partner spread a sheet over the body. He didn't look at Dr. Hoffman but drew a notebook from his pocket. "Fair's only been open—what, a week? Ten days? Jesus. We got a whole summer of this ahead?" He made a notation of some kind in his book. "You see what happened?"

"No one seems to know what happened," Dr. Hoffman said. The cop shrugged.

Dr. Hoffman looked down at his hands; his failure to help the boy who had died suddenly felt like a terrible complicity.

His hands were covered with blood. He took his handkerchief from his pocket, wiped his fingers carefully. Then he knelt beside the boy one more time and took a final, careful look at what remained visible of the body outside the fall of the sheet: the shoes, one lace untied and dangling; the narrow, delicate wrists and long fingers; the reservoir of blood filling the street with an animal smell. Why did he need an inventory of this dead boy, this unlucky, unlucky boy? He could not have said.

When he looked up, he thought he might see the fan dancer again, that she would be standing over him the way she had before. But there was no one looking at him now. The few people left standing there were looking at the body.

He stood up and walked away.

As he turned away from the young man's body, from the policeman sinking with difficulty to one knee beside it in order to search the pockets, find a name, call the survivors, break the news, Dr. Hoffman's foot struck something, and he stumbled.

He had stepped on something, he saw, bending over— a package, something infinitely hollow, which gave way under his heel with a crack. He looked, reached down for it, and then stopped.

It was a hatbox.

Dr. Hoffman stood very still, not looking at it now, simply allowing the fact of the hatbox to make itself felt.

What had Alice said? That the boy who'd brought the baby had been young and redheaded. That he'd had something happen to his face. That he'd been unlucky. Had she said that?

Or had he only added that now because he knew it was true?

He took off his glasses and held them in his hand a moment. Then he put them back on.

He looked away down the street.

The implications of this, the empty hatbox on the street by his foot, the implications for the baby, for the mother, for the young man himself, even for Dr. Hoffman—they were almost too many to consider.

Everywhere awnings were being rolled up, umbrellas furled, people were disappearing into doors, around corners, windows were snapped down. The street was almost empty; the last wave of a waiter's white cloth whisked over a table and was gone into a dark sleeve.

A streetlight flickered overhead, popped with a faraway explosion of blue sparks, went out. Darkness descended on the street.

Dr. Hoffman stood there a long time, squinting into the shadows.

And then at last he leaned over and picked up the hatbox.

Of course, it weighed nothing at all.

FIVE

S t. Louis always woke up at the same point in the
dream: a lion, its torn mane singed with fire,
burst from the smoke-filled darkness behind the flaming gates
of Creation at Coney Island's Dreamland amusement park, appearing suddenly among a crowd of horrified onlookers, shaking its heavy head from side to side in pain and bewilderment.
In every version of this dream over the past twenty years, and
there had been dozens, St. Louis woke up when the animal
turned its slow gaze on him. He woke up every time, just
at this point. The lion's stare—the accusation and danger it
contained—was too terrible to be borne, even in his sleep.

He sat up in his hammock, the rope hammock he'd made for
himself during his hours of boredom before the fair opened,
sitting cross-legged on the pier and watching the boats on Lake
Michigan. He could have slept at the Lido; there was a room
for him there, across from Caro's dressing room, that he used
when it rained. But the room's little window reminded him of a
prison cell (though he'd never been to prison) and it was too hot

in any case, even with the fan blowing from Caro's dressing room. He preferred the hammock, which he had strung in the alley behind the Café de la Paix from the deep overhang of the café's roof; the muffled sound of people talking and laughing in the street, the occasional snatches of song he recognized, the smells from the kitchen at the café—he found all these comforting. From the gutter over his head he'd tied some of Caro's paper snowflakes—delicate constructions she cut with scissors from colored bits of scrap paper or newspaper and strung on lengths of invisible black thread.

"I like to keep my hands busy—so they don't make trouble," she'd said once, giving him a significant look—she didn't approve of his habit of picking the occasional pocket. He didn't really approve of it, either; he made up for this feeling of guilt by refusing ever to steal anything from a woman and by liberating only wallets that belonged to men who distinguished themselves by being unpleasant in some way. On the train to Chicago, he had stolen the billfold of a pompous, inebriated young man who'd had the gall to empty a full martini glass onto the trembling tray of a waiter in the dining car. "I *said* no olive!" he'd declared.

Ten minutes later, St. Louis had created a disturbance by crawling under the tables, allegedly in search of his lost pet rat, and removed not only the man's wallet from his jacket pocket but also his cigarettes and an expensive-looking silver lighter.

Sitting across from Caro later that evening on the train, he watched the confetti cut from her paper fall to the ground. She'd been making him suffer in silence after the ruckus he'd created in the dining car.

"You're making a mess," he'd pointed out. But the sight of Caro, hunched over in her seat, her tongue between her teeth,

tiny bits of paper scattered over her dress and shoes and litter-
ing the floor around her feet, had moved him.

He looked up now and puffed a breath toward the paper
snowflakes. They shifted slightly, turning.

But it wasn't just the dream that had woken him. There was
noise in the street: the bells of an ambulance. The sound flew
in tight circles over the walls of the alley in which he'd strung
his hammock, over the trash cans and the short flight of
wooden steps leading to the back door of the café's kitchen,
over the upside-down gray head of the mop souring on the railing of the porch, its pose that of something flung backward and
left for dead.

What had happened out there in the street? Something.

Once there would have been a time when he could not have
passed up the commotion—what could it be now? Petty thief
apprehended? Drunken brawl in which the stumbling partici-
pants swung wide of each other and spat ridiculous insults?
Their outrage always amused St. Louis. Two women clawing
furiously at each other's dresses? But the impulse to be a spec-
tator in this disordered human theater had become gruesome
to him—what *was* it after all but laughter in the face of someone else's misfortune or humiliation? Ever since arriving in
Chicago a few weeks before, the whole endeavor of the fair—
and his life, by association—had come to seem desperate to
him. People felt cowed by what they were seeing; they could
not understand it, or they were afraid of it.

He'd seen people duck as General Italo Balbo's flyers went
overhead.

"Order a car in the morning, help in its assembly, and drive
it away the same evening!" promised a souvenir guide.

Visit the House of Tomorrow—with air-conditioning!

Stop by the model poultry farm, where the chickens lay

record numbers of eggs! See the white leghorn Lady Dixiana, 342 eggs in 365 days!

It was, he thought, simply too much gratification to be borne: Have anything in the world! Have whatever you want! Have more! People couldn't imagine all the things in store for them. General Electric understood the dark element of mystery inherent in so many inventions and innovations—it called its exhibit space the Hall of Magic, and people fell under its spell as though electricity were not a force of nature but a necromantic art.

The sound of the commotion out in the street made him depressed. What was to be seen there? What had he learned in all his years of observing people—and watching them watch other people? He could not say. But he understood that it was the only education he could have had—an education in the only world available to him, this one of carnivals and fairs and the back entrances of theaters—and he did not blame himself for this. As a young child he had believed what children are told—that they could become anything they chose; that life was just a matter of picking a label and affixing it to your shirt: pilot, letter carrier, professor, surgeon. But at some point, he could not say exactly when, he had realized that he would never become any of those things. He became, instead, a man constantly in the grip of shifting identities and masks: With a piece of charcoal he drew a straight line between his brows and pawed the ground like a bull. He juggled oranges swiped from the fruit vendor on the corner and then gave the enraged grocer a ten-dollar bill and a kiss on the forehead. He sat on the steps of city churches with a paper bag full of bread and let the pigeons collect on his shoes and sit on his hat. He did the backstroke and the crawl and the butterfly across busy intersections, horns blaring.

For what was a man like him to do? He was not freakish enough to be a medical curiosity; no one would pay money to see him. Yet he was too ugly for common society. He was good for menial tasks, for rough labor. He had become surprisingly strong for a man so small.

He closed his eyes. There would be nothing but tragedy or foolishness out there in the street, he thought. And perhaps now, after all these years, he had come inexplicably to the end of his taste for such things, though maybe taste was not the right word. Once he had *needed* to be watchful in the world, to be clever, and he had sensed correctly that there were things to be learned that only misfortune and stupidity could tell him. But he had seen enough of that now. He no longer wanted to watch people behaving badly or foolishly. Even Caro's admirers, the young men who stood up and whistled and hooted, their faces flushed—he no longer felt amused by them.

He felt sorry for them and ashamed of them and himself.

So what was next? That was the question—what was next?

For the time being, at least, there wasn't any use in lying back down and trying to fall asleep again. He rolled over in the hammock, aware of how tired he was. But the dream would only pick up where it had left off, or else simply start in all over again, a terrible retelling of the night Coney Island's biggest amusement park burned to the ground. St. Louis had been there for the fire; the spectacle had been so tragic and terrifying, and yet so beautiful, so theatrically lavish, that it had fueled over two decades' worth of his nightmares. He was sure many other bystanders that night had found their sleep likewise disturbed in the years to follow. You never forgot a thing like that.

But tonight's dream had incorporated a new element from the day's events; it did that sometimes, folding up past and present, time like a coil around which you encountered yourself again and again, unable to extricate yourself from the endless pattern of sameness.

In the dream tonight he'd been carrying a hatbox.

The Coney Island dream was so familiar he scarcely bothered to think about it much anymore. But the hatbox—that had come from the boy he'd seen earlier in the day, the one who'd wanted to know where the incubator babies were. Could he *really* have had a baby in that box? Would a man do such a thing?

In the dream, St. Louis himself had been carrying the hatbox; the boy was nowhere in sight. And he'd felt—what was it? He tried to reach back into the dream, recover the exact sensation of holding that hatbox, but it was too elusive to pin down. It wasn't as if the dream in its usual form needed any improvement, anyway. It was nothing but a serial of horrors, true to the events of that horrifying night. One of Caro's first jobs had been dancing in a revue at Coney Island's Dreamland; St. Louis, who had turned twenty that summer, had amused himself by hiring on at the Surf Avenue police-barrack stables, where he shoveled manure and cleaned tack and groomed the horses for the cops who patrolled the amusement park on horseback. He liked the big animals, their sweet breath and velvet noses, and he enjoyed practicing the occasional petty thievery—whisking full plates of sausage and sauerkraut from outdoor restaurant tables when he was hungry, picking the pockets of the gamblers and their shills—all while under the employ of the police department. As such lives go, he supposed, it was a fine enough one.

But one night in May, a fire broke out. It was started, they discovered later, by the boiling tar used by workmen in the Hell Gate show—the stuff was so hot it ignited the walls of the buildings nearby. The whole place, from Surf Avenue and the ocean to Sheridan's Walk and the new municipal bathhouse on the east, took less than four hours to burn to the ground. St. Louis, along with everyone else, could only stand by, shielding his eyes against the blistering heat, and watch.

In his dream, images from that night came before his sleeping mind in a grave and relentless procession: the animal trainers, pale and sweating in their loosely belted white jackets, lining up their pistols in the smoke-filled chaos of the night and shooting the delicate leopards as they hissed and pawed in their cages, felling the staggering elephants, felling the gigantic, rearing Clydesdales, their white eyes rolling.

He saw again the lattice of the Dreamland tower aflame, a sharp etching of gold fire against the night sky.

He saw a river of flames run down the New Iron Pier Walk, scattering the skirted gypsies and insomniac fortune-tellers, who ran screaming hither and thither before it, their belongings heaped upon their backs. Flames took down in a mouthful the shabby cabins of curio dealers and Hit-the-Nigger shacks, souvenir booths so thick with yearly applications of shiny paint that they exploded in an instant. Hot dog and ice cream vendors' carts, their bells ringing wildly, were swallowed in a wave of fire. The triple-decked carousel El Dorado, the American flag atop Abe Lent's hotel, the shifting winds carrying twisters of sparks and cyclones of burning embers across the fragile, temporary, hallucinatory landscape of Dreamland —it seemed too strange to be true, but he had seen it with his own eyes.

The nightmare was rarely content with the events exactly as

they'd occurred, though. Sometimes St. Louis found himself, in a sanguine humor that he knew with dread was only a false relief, on the cool, breeze-filled deck of the Santa Anna or the La Lorraine, the passenger ferries that brought people to Coney Island. From there he watched the fire scene from a distance, only to have enormous balls of flame suddenly tear loose from the powerful conflagration onshore and race across the black water toward the boats. And sometimes he found himself huddled on the swaying wooden ship that took hysterical passengers at Luna Park on a simulated trip to the moon; the girls hired to pose as "moon maidens" raked his face with their cold fingers, and the lagoons beneath the railing filled with the leaping reflection of flames.

Sometimes in the dream he lay injured and immobile beneath the face of the massive plaster devil who inclined himself like a hypnotic serpent over the gate to Hell.

Sometimes he ran through the Streets of Delhi, where flames leaped like swords from the rubies buried in the navels of the dancing girls.

And sometimes he whirled, sick at heart, within the Barrel of Love, his mouth forced upon the four breasts of the Siamese twins, all of them reeking of smoke and tar.

And then the dream would arrive at the lion bounding through its circle of flame, and St. Louis would wake up. If he were unlucky enough to fall back asleep, he knew he could expect to have the whole dream start all over again, frame by frame. It was better just to get up.

He dropped his leg over the side of the hammock and pushed off, setting the hammock swinging. By craning over, he could check the back door of the Café de la Paix; if it was around midnight, the back door would still be open. Though he didn't need the money, he'd picked up extra work washing glasses at the café, in addition to what he did for Caro— sweeping out the theater between her shows, taking tickets sometimes, running off her more persistent admirers, handling the books. Some nights, instead of going to Caro's show, he would go over to the café and take his place beside the other dishwashers, standing on a painted stool to reach the high metal sink comfortably. He had a talent for domestic chores; bare to the waist, his barrel chest swelling and a cloth tied around his forehead, he would make extravagant castles of lather, deep and white and luxurious as goose down. He would soap the plates and glasses, fitting the stems of wineglasses between his fingers like a juggler, turning them under the tap, and flinging the drops of water over his shoulder, where they sizzled against the still-hot surfaces of the kitchen. The closing waiters, drifting into the kitchen with the last of the dirty dishes, might share a late-night meal with him, leftover bread and onion soup and German chocolate cake. They'd look at the papers together—read about the fights (Jack Dempsey had married Hannah Williams that summer) or which rich American society girl had gotten herself engaged to which European count or prince. He hadn't gone tonight, though, too tired to stay for Caro's last show of the evening, let alone wash dishes. Still, he could usually tell the time by what was happening at the café; tonight the door was still open, a warm yellow rectangle of light, but the kitchen was quiet. They were sweeping the carpets up front, he thought. It must have been close to one.

He sat up and reached for his shoes. He would go for a walk; the fair would be mostly emptied out now. Caro's fan-dancing act and the Streets of Paris were the last attractions to stay open. Yet the heat was still staggering—unnatural and sickening and close. Pushing aside the torn bamboo screen that afforded him some privacy in his hammock, he stepped into the narrow alley that ran between the café and the streaked side wall of the Lido theater.

St. Louis had occasionally come upon prostitutes in the alley, servicing men who leaned, tense and tormented, against the walls while the girls knelt at their feet. He'd prevented what he was sure would have been a stabbing once, simply by appearing suddenly from behind his bamboo screen, scratching his scalp; three young men and a glinting knife had scattered. And more than once he'd seen bills changing hands between violent-looking men with three days of beard on their jaws, their hats pulled low over their eyes. Yet he imagined that he himself did not excite much interest, let alone fear, in those he passed; it was only the surprise of him, coming out of nowhere. Though his head was certainly too large for his body, it was not so large as to be immediately grotesque, the material creature of a nightmare. He fell instead into that nameless category between man and freak, neither one nor the other—*simply ugly,* he told himself—and so imagined himself in some fashion invisible, like a creature one has no name for and so cannot recall once it has passed from view. Caro said it was the head of a wise man.

"Don't you know," she told him, "that the saints were the homeliest kind of people?"

St. Louis didn't think she was right. Why should the saints, as a group, be uglier than the rest of mankind?

But Caro swore it was true. "Everybody knows that," she said airily. "You see it all the time."

St. Louis turned out of the alley into the street. The ambulance had driven off. There were a few people over by the steps of the Lido, standing close together under the streetlamps, talking about something of mutual interest. A cigarette girl, in

high heels and fishnet stockings, leaned against the wall of the
theater, her hands draped loosely over the edge of her tray, her
eyes closed. But no one was sitting at the outdoor café across
the street—and it usually stayed open to catch the crowds
from Caro's last show. Instead, the waiters were standing close
together just inside the French doors in a hushed and watchful
way, behind the pleats of muslin curtains, the funeral black of
their jackets melting away beneath their pale faces and the
shiny, parted wings of their dark hair.

Something was wrong, St. Louis thought. Something bad
had happened here.

And then he saw the baby doctor.

Hoffman—it was Dr. Hoffman.

He was sitting on the curb under a streetlight. Was he drunk?
St. Louis stopped and stared. Hoffman had the look of too
much liquor about him—black hair disheveled, a shoelace
untied, his shirt untucked, his expression dull. He sat there on
the curb like a child, staring straight ahead. He looked so
young that St. Louis was struck by the foolishness of Hoffman's
mustache. It looked like one of the false mustaches made of
felt that children use to play pirate.

The entrance to the alley was less than fifty feet from
Hoffman. St. Louis watched the doctor for a moment and then
began to move slowly toward him. Could Hoffman really be
drunk? It was impossible. The baby doctor? Soused?

He walked carefully, slowly; he made no noise, and he kept
his eyes on Hoffman the whole time, as if the doctor might suddenly jump up and run off if alarmed. But as he drew nearer,
he saw that Hoffman was not drunk. The expression St. Louis
had detected on his face was not dullness but a kind of tired
devastation. Quietly, St. Louis crossed the street so as to be
able to get a better look at him. If this baby doctor, this famous

baby doctor, was sitting on a street corner, something was very wrong.

He moved slowly toward Hoffman, keeping his eyes on him, but the doctor did not seem to notice St. Louis's approach. He sat inordinately still, his knees and feet pressed close together. When Hoffman shifted a little, reached back to withdraw a handkerchief from his pocket, and began to raise it to his forehead, St. Louis stopped, not wanting to come any closer. Under the queer artificial light of the electric streetlamp, St. Louis saw that the handkerchief was badly stained. At almost the same moment, Hoffman, too, seemed to remember that the handkerchief was soiled and carefully put it away again.

On the far side of the street, the cigarette girl pushed away from the wall of the Lido with an obvious effort and stalked slowly past them, her eyes averted, her shadow falling across the cobblestones and licking the toe of Hoffman's shoe. The group of people in front of the Lido had vanished as if they had turned to smoke. Was he seeing things? Hadn't they been there a moment ago?

St. Louis took a few steps closer, and when he was almost level with Hoffman, a few feet before coming into the doctor's unwavering line of vision, he stopped. He did not know what to do, and then, more surprisingly, he realized that he felt some urgency to remove Hoffman from his place on the curb—it didn't look good, the baby doctor sitting in the filth of the street. But it was more than that. This man—for whatever it was worth—was responsible for all those babies, all those tiny little helpless babies. He ought not to be sitting here like this, looking so ruined. It was—irresponsible. It was derelict.

Yet what business was it of his? This was a question he could not answer. Nor could he ignore the impulse to get Hoffman out of the street.

After another moment's hesitation, he stepped forward briskly into the pool of light at Hoffman's feet.

Hoffman looked up at him, not surprised to see him, but as if he had expected it, expected someone to come and lead him away.

And then St. Louis saw the hatbox.

It sat on the sidewalk beside Hoffman. It was a plain hatbox, pale gray, decorated with garlands of tiny blue and pink flowers, a black lid. Common enough. One side of the box had been dented and crumpled. St. Louis could see that someone had made an effort to straighten it out, restore its original shape. A kind of freezing stillness settled over his limbs.

That was the young man's hatbox.

St. Louis had thought there wasn't anything left that could shock him. After all, who could top his own private tally of witnessed misery? Pipo and Zipo, the microcephalics at Coney Island; the fat girl who sang the "Bumble Bee Stomp" until people nearly wet themselves with laughter . . . oh, God, he could go on and on. That was the problem. But this—for now he felt sure there had been a baby in the hatbox; why else would Hoffman have it with him now?—this had the force of the unimaginable.

"Excuse me," Hoffman said politely. "May I help you?"

He sounded exactly like a drunken man, the same elaborate and comically precise formality in his speech. But no, Hoffman was not drunk. St. Louis felt himself held under Hoffman's regard for a moment and then, picking up the hatbox carefully, the doctor stood up.

"Good evening," Hoffman said, equally carefully.

And then he was gone, walking slowly down the center of the empty street, the pools of light like stones across a river, back toward the baby house, the hatbox under his arm. And yet St. Louis felt that Hoffman had not really seen him; he would not remember this exchange in the morning. The street was entirely deserted now; even the cigarette girl had disappeared as if she had ascended up a tiring flight of steps into the sky. A blue smoke, like the puffs sent out from the bellows at the start of Caro's act, filled the air under the hissing streetlights. But he was not entirely alone; he thought he could make out, standing behind the muslin curtains of the French doors of the café, a quartet of waiters staring out at him, partly concealed. Their faces were indistinct as clay; their arms hung limply at their sides. St. Louis had to look twice to be sure they were real, not just wooden forms propped up in front of the doors to give the illusion of activity inside. From far away, he heard a lion roar; that would be Queenie or Brutus, St. Louis told himself, turning around hopelessly in the street as if to face the lions freed from captivity. *I have seen them in the Lion Motordrome,* he thought. *They are real.*

But there was nothing there. There was just Hoffman, pacing off the distance between them carefully, never looking back, the empty hatbox under his arm.

St. Louis headed away from Lake Michigan and toward the long lagoon that ran north to south down the center of the fairgrounds. Lake Michigan was too large for him at night, especially this night, too endless and too deep; its vague, low, far-off sounds were mournful and strange. He steered instead toward the lagoon, along the shoreline dotted with the obedient moorings of empty paddleboats and serene flocks of ducks. It was a tame place, full now of cool, ashy shadows under a heavy moon, the sinking planet's edges indistinct. The grass was mowed closely here; the willows' fronds rustled. A pagoda could be seen alone on the far shore.

He came to the walkway that ran along the lagoon. The heat of the day had lifted here by the water; coolness hovered in the air. In a few hours, he judged, the sun would be up, and the baking heat would settle again over the taut cables of the suspension bridge, the monumental buildings of the fair, its minarets and towers, its tricks and wonders and games of chance. Chicago's new skyscrapers would loom in the background through the haze, lofty and insubstantial.

He walked along in the pools of shadows thrown by the slender young willows planted every few yards along the water's edge. Crossing the wide strip of grass that separated the path from the water, he sat down at the shoreline, took off his shoes, and dipped his feet into the water. He'd never had a really good pair of shoes, not a pair that fit him right, and his feet were often sore. It seemed almost inexplicable to him, unlacing his shoes now, that a thing as simple as a well-fitting pair of shoes should have eluded him. After all, it wasn't as if Caro wouldn't have bought him anything he wanted. She rolled her eyes at him sometimes. "What do you want to look like a bum for?" she said. "You'd scare a person."

"That's my *job*," he'd said pointedly. "I am a bum."

"Well, you don't really scare anybody," Caro told him. "You've just got this way of talking them to death. And you could look just fine if you'd wear some decent clothes."

"The clothes do not make the man." He'd given her a haughty look, but even as he said it, he was struck by the truth, that, in his case, he *was* in fact made by what he wore—the ten-gallon hats, the too-big tuxedo jackets, the long aviator scarves and feed caps and mismatched argyle socks and earmuffs. Take them away, and what was left?

What was the point of nice clothes for a man like him? Still, shoes . . . he could have had comfortable shoes.

And then, suddenly, he was furious—at himself, at Hoffman, at the boy with the hatbox. He'd had a *baby* in a hatbox! A baby!

St. Louis put his head into his hands. And now something had happened, he thought—to the man or the baby, or maybe to both of them. Now—*now* there's a catastrophe building.

He'd felt it all along, ever since the fair opened, or even before, while it was still being built.

He sat glumly and looked down at his legs. The water was so dark he looked to himself like an amputee sitting there, his pants rolled to the knee, his legs lopped off at midcalf by the black line of water. He stirred his invisible feet, made the water wrinkle. Well. He lived in a world where people could put a baby in a hatbox and bring it to the fair. It shouldn't surprise him. Why was it surprising him? It was as if he'd never seen how ugly it all was before. And now everything—all of it—was ugly.

He had made an error, a significant error, and he was only now beginning to see it. All his restless wanderings after Caro, his inability to stray far from her side—where had they brought him?

Twenty-two years ago, Caro had left for Washington to accompany Mrs. Minnie Crane as the old woman's milliner's model for what was to have been a week, while Mrs. Crane showed her hats to ladies' clubs and private customers. Caro disappeared on Mrs. Crane the last day, leaving a note that said she was going off to seek her fame and fortune with a dancing troupe and that no one should worry about her; she'd write. St. Louis had gone after her the day after Mrs. Crane came back with the news. He had left the farmhouse well before dawn, a letter for his aunt and uncle explaining his purpose set first on his bed, then on the kitchen table, then in the center of the griddle, which lay on the stove, as if they might not notice his absence otherwise. He managed to find Caro in Washington purely by luck; he hadn't stopped to consider that he might never find her. When he got off the train at Union Station, he saw an advertisement for a new club and dancing show. Caro had probably seen the same one, he thought, and there she was when he walked in that night, last girl on the right, kicking high.

He'd been eighteen years old.

He'd been following her, more or less the whole time, ever since, traveling from city to city, fair to fair, sometimes staying on behind somewhere, telling her he'd catch up later. The weeks he'd spent away from her over the years had been filled sometimes with spells of fierce homesickness. He'd always thought that homesickness had to do with Caro herself; out of her orbit, he became untethered. And yet Caro herself was nearby now; he could go wake her up if he wanted, make her sit up in bed and talk to him. But if Caro was here, what was this sudden, penetrating longing? Why did he remember his childhood game of tracking a guinea through the shrubbery to find where she had laid her eggs? Why did he remember the long meadows full of stiff sweet grass that moved like the surface of the sea, or the rare luna moths that held against the walls of the farmhouse at night? His childhood had been full of things to touch, and he had liked to put his hands into fur and feathers, to roll an egg between his palms, to stroke the horse's flank and the dog's ear. He had liked other children, had sat in school mesmerized by them. He had even loved their various smells, like little fires that had been lit all around him in the classroom to send forth mysterious, coiling columns of scent— soap, mud, hay, apples, wind, manure, even the acid tang of sickness. He had been tormented by the long yellow braids of a girl who sat in front of him in fourth grade, had wanted to brush the silky ends of her hair against his cheek, his desire fixed and painful. He had never touched her.

Reaching down now and cupping water from the lagoon in his hands, St. Louis sniffed it. It did not smell like real water to him—not like the springwater back on the farm. The lithia waters from the farm smelled like the distillate of life itself. No, *had* smelled, he reminded himself. The spring had dried up, his uncle Warren had said. And again St. Louis felt the impact of that loss. Something intrinsic to his being had disappeared from the world.

When the spring had been discovered on the property, Warren had built an arched cover of brick and mortar for it and a small bottling house, hiring two men from town to come on Saturdays to help with the bottling and packaging. St. Louis had liked the bottling house. He'd liked haunts in general— the hollow, sour-smelling cave in the center of boxwoods planted in a ring in the circular drive that ran up to the farmhouse, the old icehouse with its mystical furnishings of spiderwebs, the space on the floor between the horsehair settee in the parlor and the dark, glass-front bookshelves, a narrow, cool place where he could lie on his stomach and read.

But his favorite place was the spring, where a thin wick of cold water was trained over a heap of small, rounded stones, an ancient font deep in a grove of white oaks, hickories, and ash.

Before the bottling house was built, St. Louis would lie on his back in the deep pile of moss beneath the spring, his mouth open wide. He would make a siphon of his hands and encourage a trickle of water to splash over his face and run under his collar, seeping down his arms and chest and belly and legs. The water was so cold, cold as the stars, he thought, the water of high altitudes, buried deep in the center of the earth.

Warren had made modest claims for his water, and physicians he'd asked to write endorsements replied by letter that they had prescribed the waters to therapeutic effect. Eventually Warren had printed up a brochure in which his lithia water was said to cure a long list of ailments: dyspepsia, Bright's disease, gout, biliousness, nervous prostration and indigestion, rheumatism and dropsy, albuminuria, piles, torpid liver, female weakness, and malaria. An etching on the pamphlet showed a mysterious figure, clad in long garments and a turban, standing by a small waterfall. A stick in his hand struck the source of the water from the rock; his other hand was held high in benediction, index finger raised prophetically.

St. Louis had once read the chemists' report on Day's Lithia Water; it contained, the report said, trace amounts of sulfuric acid and manganous carbonate; grains of sodium chloride, sodium sulfate, and potassium sulfate; calcium, bicarbonate calcium, carbon magnesium, ferrous carbonate, alumina, silica, iodine, and lithium. All these collected and pooled below ground as rainwater dissolved through the twinkling strata of the earth. But St. Louis did not care about any of it. Those were not his ailments, nor his complaints. Could ugliness, the miserable state of the orphan, be cured? It seemed to him—for a time— that the water might change him, though not in any way he could formulate clearly. He had no idea what exactly the water might do for him, but lying there in the moss, he drank deeply. And when he was old enough to understand that his incantations and religious doses had failed him, he stopped going to the spring. They drank the lithia water at the table, of course, but it wasn't the same as kneeling in the dark and cupping it into his hands. He passed beyond his desperation for things to be made right and instead made of his longing something small, which he swallowed like a tooth, its barbed root settling near his heart.

His longing for home had always been assuaged by Caro's presence; yet now it seemed to him that she was no longer enough to block that hole in his heart. He'd broached the subject with Caro directly just before the fair opened. Didn't she want to call it quits?

But Caro had been annoyed. "What are you saying?" she'd said sharply. "I'm getting old? I'm getting fat?"

He'd protested.

"You can go whenever you like," Caro had said finally.

But later she had come and found him, reading in the last row of seats in the Lido, which was empty for a few hours between shows. She'd put her arms around him, rested her head on his shoulder. "Don't leave," she whispered. "We'll go home one day; I promise."

And since she would not go home—not yet—he must be near her, for if the feeling of home could be divided in his heart, Caro held the greater half of it.

He looked up now from the shore of the lagoon, where he was still treading water, the cool relief washing up his legs.

He had worn for the last few years a set of brogues given him by a policeman at Coney Island; they'd belonged to the cop's brother, and the policeman had disbursed his dead brother's belongings among his needy friends who'd worked the amusement parks as night watchmen and bouncers.

"No good wasting 'em," the heavy-faced policeman had said quietly, standing in the center of a group of people one rainy night and passing out his dead brother's shirts and folded trousers, balled socks and soft handkerchiefs, from a bag at his feet. "Good stuff like this shouldn't go to waste." And he handed the shoes to St. Louis, who had stepped forward with the others, his hands outstretched. He'd noticed that the policeman's fingernails were bitten to the quick.

This was just a few months after the stock market crash, and no one wasted anything, not even Caro, who regarded money as something to be given away fast. St. Louis had seen sadder things happen, he'd thought at the time, fitting his feet into the shoes with a nod for the deceased man. Still, the shoes had been too large, and though he stuffed the toes with rags, they had chafed, leaving ridged calluses on his instep and heel. Why hadn't he ever gone out and bought himself a new pair? Why had he punished himself like this?

As he sat there, splashing in the lagoon's still waters, a movement on the ground beside him caught his eye. Something small and white inched slowly, noiselessly, across the grass. After a moment, St. Louis recognized it and leaned over to pick it up. It was one of the baby turtles that had become, inexplicably, the hottest souvenir of the fair that year. The turtles' tiny shells, not much bigger than a poker chip, had been enameled with a bright circle of white to resemble a seashell. A curlicue of minute red roses on a green stem had been painted in the center of the white circle. He lifted the little creature gently into the palm of his hand, watched its tiny, wizened head and legs wave a moment in protest before retracting into the shell.

He looked down at the turtle. The creature had almost made it to freedom, an escapee from the shallow bins full of filthy sand, tired ribs of celery, and wilted lettuce leaves. He tapped respectfully on the shell with one finger and then set the turtle down in the grass, where it lay perfectly still.

St. Louis waited, the concentric rings of ripples around his legs spreading out into infinite, flattening degrees across the still, dark water. After a few minutes, the turtle's scaly head emerged. St. Louis saw the black bead of its eye. Then the turtle's legs appeared and, after another few minutes of primeval patience, it began to move, bearing itself forward under the weight of its foolishly painted shell. St. Louis followed it with his eyes through the short grass until it disappeared into the darkness. After a moment, he heard a low, soft *plop* as the turtle found the water and began its weightless release into the embrace of the lagoon.

St. Louis's heart gave a minor twist, an arrhythmic pause of envy, perhaps, of admiration or even collaborative joy. What a thing, to have escaped! To have made it across the complicated, transient spaces of the fair, between wheels and menacing heels, amid the dashing of children and the shuffle of stunned, bashful farmers with their heavy, unlaced boots. To have been missed by the tumble of acrobats and the unbroken line of weaving parades, the tramping of thousands of feet and hooves, to have made it all the way to the thin, silvered line of water. If the turtle had flown, St. Louis could not have been at that moment more awed.

He twitched the stumps of his feet. He was really tired now. His eyelashes fluttered delicately shut, his mouth opened, and he imagined for a moment slipping down a canal, down the bank, and into the black envelope of water, a curtain dropping on the violent theater of the concourse, the noise of the crowd, the battery and congress of all the world around him.

Is that hatbox baby still alive? he wondered, almost asleep in the dream of his own vanishing. And who could say at that moment whether he meant the baby in the hatbox or himself, the stunted boy who'd lain on the moss beside the spring, filling his mouth with sweet water and wishing for a miracle.

But then, as the sun suddenly flew up over the edge of the

water, its carnival light rolling down the street behind him, as the ferris wheel twitched against its stays in a tunnel of wind, he thought he could at least hope for one thing: that the baby, that innocent baby, that orphan, was still alive, and that somewhere, Hoffman had him safe.

SIX

There were several deaths at the Century of Progress that summer. A man claiming to be a trained parachutist plunged to his death from an airplane scrolling in over the airfield during an afternoon air show. Around him, the other jumpers' chutes blossomed like Japanese paper flowers in water, a field of yellow and red poppies against the blue sky. But one chute failed to open, and the falling man made a small, dark mark sliding through the garden of bright balloons toward the earth and the bleachers of horrified spectators. After the accident, the man's relatives said he had been depressed; money troubles, they intimated. (Who didn't have money troubles?) But they expressed shock and dismay that he would choose to end his life in such a public, theatrical way. He had always been a quiet person, they said.

Two visitors to the fair—one a fifty-five-year-old pig farmer from Pennsylvania, the other a town selectman from Abbott, Maine—suffered heart attacks at the fair and died, one in June, the other in August. The pig farmer was touring the model homes exhibit with his wife, where they were admiring an "ironing station" cleverly built into the pantry of a pink bungalow. His wife was pointing to the hinge mechanism for the concealed ironing board. She leaned over to say to her husband, "Chester, you could make that," when he got an awful look on his face, put his hand up to cover his mouth, and then sank to his knees.

The town selectman from Maine was accompanied by his two grandsons. Their mother was in the hotel, resting; too hot for her, she had said, waving her father and little boys on without her that morning. The selectman, sixty-four years old, was watching his grandsons laugh themselves silly over the antics of two clowning pirates on the Enchanted Island who were stabbing each other over and over again through the armpit with rubber knives and falling into the water. Watching the pirates climb from the water for the hundredth time, he began to laugh and then experienced a searing, suffocating pain that radiated throughout his body. An explosion had been detonated at the base of his spine; the world was lit with a burst of light and then went suddenly dark. He slumped over against the wooden railing.

It took hours for the boys' mother to be located. The children didn't know the name of the hotel where they were staying, and the youngest, only four years old, could not be made to stop crying until he was finally handed over to his mother by an exhausted policeman who had called all the hotels in Chicago looking for her.

The death of the young man with the hatbox, the father of the baby now safely deposited in Dr. Hoffman's nursery, was the first of the summer.

The fair's backers worried that such a brutal, apparently senseless murder would cast a pall over the summer's proceedings, and they urged police to make an arrest—any arrest—quickly. And yet, though some had worried that the murder would be a bad omen, would scare people away from the Streets of Paris, the affair disappeared in the public consciousness almost instantly. Police never made an arrest in the case, but that didn't seem to trouble anyone. No one imagined that a killer was on the loose, someone who might strike again. No one felt threatened. It was as if, in fact, the young man and his murderer had never really existed or had appeared on the scene for the duration of their brief, tragic, violent collision, only to fade away almost instantly, out of the world altogether. Even people who were witnessses, who'd been to see Caro Day dance that same night, at that same show, later found that they could not clearly recall what had happened. People remembered Caro herself; they never forgot their first sight of her, dancing across the stage and glowing as if she had been dipped in the sunset. But the events afterward were shrouded in a thick mist. There was no agreement about the victim, either, the young man—whether he had struck his assailant first, or whether he was big, or small, or dark haired, or blond. The murderer? He had been a Negro. A white man. He was young, or old. A man with a scar. Or a limp. They had exchanged angry words, or none at all. There had been a crowd, some sort of struggle.

It had been so hot, they would say, passing a hand over their foreheads. So very hot.

The young man's wife—silly, sentimental, devastated Sylvie. Told of her young husband's death, she became insensible. Her sister was called.

And the baby? The baby? What happened to the baby, Evie wanted to know, weeping, laying her hands over Sylvie's empty belly.

Sylvie told her the baby had died.

Evie was bewildered. Died? When? When had it been born? What was he doing at the fair? she asked Sylvie. When had this happened?

"How should I know? How should I know?" Sylvie cried. "Who told him where to go? Not me!"

How could she say that it had all frightened her to death? The labor, the birth, the half-dead infant that did not look like any baby she'd ever seen. The baby's birth, her husband's death— they were linked up in her mind now like evil charms. "It was born too soon," she said at last, in a dull voice. "He'd gone to take it to the doctor, the one you told us about, at the fair."

Evie clapped a hand over her mouth.

Mrs. Hermann, embarrassed in front of this pretty, clever girl—she knew Evie was a schoolteacher—hung her head over Sylvie's feet, which she was massaging with wet towels. Mrs. Hermann was exhausted. She had been awake so long now, first delivering the baby and then staying with Sylvie while her husband went off to the fair, and later answering the door when the policeman came, his hat in his hand, in the middle of the night. She was ashamed—perhaps she should never have sent him to that baby doctor. And yet she was angry, too, for she felt some suggestion of blame in the air. Evie was plainly horrified at all that had transpired in the dingy apartment in just twenty-four hours. Mrs. Hermann wanted to defend herself; she had done her best, she wanted to say. She had delivered plenty of babies. Taking that poor wee creature to the baby doctor at the fair—it had been a *good* idea, the only thing to be done.

But Evie, sitting on a straight chair by Sylvie's bed, stared back and forth between the two of them as if they were mad.

She would have to leave in a few minutes; school began at eight. She looked out the window onto the fire escape, to two pale blue dishcloths hanging stiffly over the black iron bars where they had been set out to dry. "He took the baby to the fair," she repeated at last in a whisper.

Mrs. Hermann hung her head. "It wouldn't live," she said. "It wasn't going to live. *It was too small.* Only he could help it."

Evie moved over to sit down on the bed, put her arms around her sister. "Sylvie," she said, "I will go there and see, see if he—"

But Sylvie struggled up in bed beside her. "No!" She reached for her sister's arm with hot, urgent fingers. Her pretty face was torn with red welts from scratching herself during the labor; the shape of her round cheeks was distorted from weeping.

A thunderstorm was blowing up outside. Evie could smell Lake Michigan the way she always could when it was about to rain. She looked down at her sister, horrified at her, ashamed of her, and yet full of pity at the same time.

"Just leave it now," Sylvie said to her, falling back against the pillow, exhausted. "It's all over. It's dead; I know it is. I saw it, Evie. You didn't, you didn't see it." And she burst into a fresh bout of weeping. "It was . . . terrible."

Mrs. Hermann listened to all this, bathing feverish Sylvie's forehead, her feet, her legs. She held her tongue now, deeply shocked by the news of the young man's murder, by all the events of the last twenty-four hours. It was none of her business, none of her business.

At last, collecting herself, brushing her hands down her skirt, Evie thanked Mrs. Hermann, kissed her cheek with what seemed to Mrs. Hermann surprising feeling, and sent her home with a quarter of a pound cake she had baked the night before. Mrs. Hermann opened the door to her own apartment at last, deeply troubled, and came heavily to her knees beside her own bed after almost twenty-four hours without sleep.

What had happened to the poor baby? she wondered. She would pray for it, in any case, whether it be here on this earth still or up in heaven. She had never seen a baby so small. She thought Sylvie was probably right—that it had died. But the young man hadn't had it with him when he was, when he was—but she had to veer away in her mind from the violence of what had happened to the young man, that nice young man. At least, she thought, no one had *mentioned* a baby. Surely they would have mentioned a baby, if one had been found.

And Sylvie hadn't asked, either. Mrs. Hermann had watched Sylvie's face, watched her eyes, when the policeman, an older man with a distracting brown birthmark in the shape of a small cloud above his right eye, came to stand awkwardly by the bed, his hat in his hand. And why would the policeman ask about a baby unless they'd found one? The policeman wouldn't know anything, except maybe that Sylvie had been ill; she certainly looked ill, lying there in the bed, and what was there to suggest a baby had been born? Mrs. Hermann had watched Sylvie's eyes, wide and horrified, slide away from Mrs. Hermann's face. And she'd understood then that Sylvie would not say anything about the baby.

Kneeling by her own bed, Mrs. Hermann tried to understand this, tried to understand the sense of guilt she felt now. Oughtn't she to have asked the policeman herself, later, quietly, at the door when she saw him out? Oughtn't she to have explained? But it was as if by not mentioning it, she and Sylvie could, together, simply erase the whole terrible night. Now there was a hole in the world that was quickly being sealed over with the future itself, a dense wall of clouded glass. Their

grief, though surely Sylvie held the greater share of it—over
the baby's disappearance, over Sylvie's husband's terrible murder—could be held at bay by Mrs. Hermann and Sylvie's col-
lusion. It would stand awhile, she knew, a dark thing in the
corner, and then gradually fade from sight. Sylvie was young,
after all, Mrs. Hermann thought. And pretty. There'd be another husband before too long, another child. This would all be
in the past and forgotten.

Mrs. Hermann closed her eyes and folded her hands. If the
baby was with the doctor, if his father had managed to get him
there, then that was all that could be done now by any of them.
Maybe later, when she felt better, Sylvie could decide what to
do. Though Mrs. Hermann did not think Sylvie would go and
claim her child, if her child still lived. Mrs. Hermann put her
forehead onto her curled fingers, closed her eyes. He hadn't
had it with him when . . . Maybe he'd gotten it to the doctor
before—maybe. The room swam before her, God's hand delib-
erating over her head. She was so tired now.

I did the best I could, the best I knew how, she thought.

Rest their souls, she prayed. *God rest their souls.*

Evie taught school in a daze. There was only a week left
of classes, and she worried about what would happen to her
pupils over the long summer vacation. She was more than usually
tender with the children, particularly the younger ones, many of
whom looked especially poor and underfed to her that day; she
put little squares of pound cake into their hands at the lunch
hour, touched their heads. Sitting in the hard chair by her desk,
framed by the big map of the world hanging behind her, she had
the children come up one at a time to tell her their sums so she
could smile at each individually, concentrate on their faces, their
hands, their clothes, the irrefutable presence of them.

Before going back to Sylvie's apartment that evening, she went home briefly to her room, where she exchanged her blouse for a clean one, rinsed out the one she had worn during the day, and left it hanging over a chair by the window. Her landlady, who'd roused her earlier that morning when the police had called, closed her own door with a soft click when Evie went back downstairs. People hated bad news, Evie thought. The woman wasn't unkind, but she would not want to be mixed up in anything that involved a telephone call from the police at five in the morning.

Evie stepped out into the early-evening air; the street was full of children, playing hopscotch and jacks on the sidewalk, and young mothers, sitting in twos and threes on the steps, smoking cigarettes and talking. She would buy some sausage on the way to Sylvie's, she thought, stepping carefully over a game of jacks, and some apples if she could find any. They needed to eat, both of them.

Sylvie had an appetite. She ate not only her sausage but half of Evie's, too, shuddering with weakness. Evie cleared away the plate and came back to Sylvie's bedside with a knife and cored the apples onto her handkerchief, which she had spread over the sheet. She would have liked tea, but there was only a little coffee in the kitchen, so she made two weak cups and sweetened them with a lump of brown sugar she found hardened in a little red bowl. Where had Sylvie gotten such a pretty thing? She looked at her sister, who was lying back against the pillows, the cup of coffee at her lips, her eyes closed. She felt angry with her, almost too angry to speak—appalled and bewildered by her attitude about the baby, her apparent lack of feeling for Jack himself. Jack! Evie was suddenly aware that her brother-in-law's name would not be spoken now more than a dozen or more times before they ceased to speak of him at all.

And yet her anger at Sylvie was complicated by her pity. She had thought Sylvie lucky to have been married, but too young. Sylvie was spoiled, in a way; she could work hard, for she was young and strong, but she wanted disproportionate rewards for that work—pretty clothes and meals out and entertainment—more often than Evie thought was reasonable. Unmarried herself, and at thirty almost ten years Sylvie's senior, she had worried about the marriage from the start. But Jack was—Jack *had been,* she corrected herself, with another sickening sensation of loss, one in a series of the quickly moving waves that crashed over her—a kind boy. He had loved Sylvie so much, with such open adoration. But Sylvie had only liked the thought of marriage, Evie suspected, the idea of setting up house, someone to provide for her. And yet surely she was heartbroken now?

Evie looked at her sister's body, a body that had so recently, so miraculously, transformed itself into the notion of motherhood. And yet that's all it was: a notion. One day there'd been a swelling under Sylvie's skin, a life waiting to happen, this enormous gift, thought Evie. And then the next day, nothing. Not even a trace of a baby or the man who had fathered it. It was baffling. It was as if they'd all dreamed it.

The room was growing dark, full of dusk and shadows. An apologetic grayness had settled over the room's few furnishings—the bed with Sylvie's body beneath the sheet, two straight-backed chairs, the queer pedestal table with a dark green felt cloth over it, a trunk with brass fittings. How little Sylvie and Jack seemed to have done to make this a home, she thought. Perhaps Sylvie had no instinct for it, after all, though she always dressed stylishly. Evie stood up and paced the little room. A shirt of Jacks, soiled and sour smelling, rust-colored blood on the front, was balled up in a corner. Evie stooped to pick it up, held it wonderingly.

She did not want to blame Sylvie now, but she felt it absolutely necessary to make her see that they must make inquiries at the fair. She felt she could persuade Sylvie to let her go and ask about the baby.

"Sylvie," Evie began from the far side of the room, as gently as she could. "You've lost a husband, but perhaps you still have a child. Your own child!"

Sylvie made no response, lying with her face turned away toward the wall.

"Doesn't that move you?" Evie tried to control her impatience. "Don't you want to know what's happened to him?"

But Sylvie was even more adamant than she had been earlier, though with a sulkiness that made Evie want to slap her. "I know what happened," Sylvie said, sliding down in the bed under the sheet. "It died. I know it did."

Evie slowly folded Jack's shirt and put it down on a chair. She would take it home and wash it, she said to herself, trying to stifle her feeling of rage. Then she returned to the bed and sat down at Sylvie's feet. She was more troubled than she could have imagined at the thought of the baby—this relation of hers, her own nephew—somehow adrift in the world. Or if not adrift, then . . . "You ought to find out," she said bluntly. "So that there can be a service, at least." She paused. Sylvie had said nothing about a funeral for Jack. "Just like for his father."

Sylvie sat up in bed suddenly. "What does it *matter?*" she cried, clutching the sheet. "What do you know about *any* of it, Evie? It's my life! It's happened, and now it's over. All of it!" She looked regretful, close to tears again, and Evie's heart was moved. "I haven't got any of them now!" Sylvie went on. "They've all been taken away. And I couldn't keep a baby by myself. What would I do for money? I haven't even got a job anymore!"

Evie began to interrupt. This was silly! Lots of women had babies alone, though not by choice, of course. "We could care for it together," she started. "I could—"

Sylvie cut her off; her tone was knowing and definite. Evie suddenly had the feeling that Sylvie had lain in bed all day soberly considering her options, her future.

"It isn't alive," Sylvie said now. "Really and truly, Evie. I know it. God has just taken away my whole past. It wasn't meant to be. None of it."

Evie flinched at the mention of God. Sylvie had no right to bring up God; it was calculated and despicable of her. She didn't even pretend to believe in God otherwise.

Evie felt a sharp distaste for her sister now that bordered on disgust. How could Sylvie just let it go like that? It was shocking. She regarded Sylvie's face now. Sylvie lay with one arm thrown back over her eyes. There was a trace of grease glowing on her cheek in the darkness, from the sausage. Evie stood up again and walked to the other side of the bed, to the window, where she could look out. She couldn't see the fair from here, but she knew it was there, a quivering place of sound and smells and streaking light at the edge of the lake. The whole city was grateful for the fair, for the money it brought to town. She had ridden the Ferris wheel on her one afternoon there. At the top of the wheel, she had looked out over the fair from the gently swinging car and had thought that, from high above, the fairgrounds looked like something in the picture books she read to her children at school, a magical lost city hidden in a dark valley, a brightly painted scene made of little dabs of color from a paint box. Suspended high in the sky on the Ferris wheel, she'd listened as the cacophony of the fair drained away to a barely audible hum, a tinkling of musical notes beneath the sound of the wind.

At school, sitting with her children in the afternoons after
lunch, she let them run their hands over the pretty pictures in
the books, as if the scenes of castles and oceans and mountains and deserts and faraway countries were something you
could feel in the tips of your fingers, little worlds under a spell,
all the people sleeping, the horses stalled in the meadows with
their noses in the emerald grass, cars pausing endlessly at intersections, a woman leaning from a tiny window and calling
down into a street where everyone had turned to stone.

"Promise me, Evie," Sylvie said from behind her.

Evie turned around.

Sylvie was sitting straight up in bed, the sheet held to her
breasts. She looked drained and exhausted. "Promise me you
won't go there and look for him," Sylvie said again. "I . . . I
couldn't bear it." She began to weep. "Promise," she said.
"Promise, promise."

Evie didn't want to, but the voice would not stop. *Promise,
promise, promise.*

"Don't." Evie came back to the bed and sat down awkwardly
to put her arms around Sylvie. "Stop now. It's all right; I won't."

"Promise," said Sylvie again. This pact between them, the
pact of children, was all that was needed. She looked up at
Evie, her face a ruin.

"Yes," Evie said. "All right. I promise."

There was nothing to do in the small room. Evie offered to read to her, but Sylvie said no, she wanted to try to
sleep. If only her breasts didn't hurt so much. "I feel like I'm
going to burst," she moaned.

Evie retrieved the dishcloths from the fire escape and wet
them with cool water. Sylvie lay in bed, the cloths across her
chest, and reached for Evie's hand. "Don't leave," she begged,

drawing her sister close in the darkness of the room. "I just know I'm going to have bad dreams. I know I am, about Jack, and—"

"Shh." Evie did not want to think about Jack, about what had happened to him. And yet she wanted to ask Sylvie more about what the police had said. Why would someone have killed Jack? Of all the people likely to cause trouble in the world, she thought, Jack was as shy of confrontation as anyone she'd ever known. She could not understand what had happened to him, how he could have provoked such a terrible attack. And despite herself, she could not stop thinking about the baby. She remembered her visit to the incubator exhibit; she'd marveled at the size of the babies there, a respectful, almost religious feeling coming over her as she watched the nurses move quietly around the immaculate nursery, so certain and so deft. She was used to children, but the tiny babies in the exhibit had seemed like something more than ordinary children. The care lavished on them suggested that these babies had a special destiny. Their circumstances, the hush around them, the mysterious, gleaming equipment, the handsome doctor moving from one incubator to another—all this inspired reverence in her. *How good they are,* she had thought. *How good and how clever and how brave.*

She could only hope that Jack had somehow managed to deliver his baby to the great doctor. Evie felt certain that if he had, the doctor would take the best possible care of it. But if they did not know a baby's parents, what then? She understood from her visit to the incubator exhibit that families were not charged for such care, that their children were serving the advancement of medical science. But what would become of the baby if no one ever came to claim it?

Sylvie had fallen asleep at last. Evie stood up from the chair

by the bed. She would need to sleep if she was to be good for
anything in the morning. She pulled her shirt loose from the
waist of her skirt and slipped off her shoes. *Forgive me*, she
thought, looking down at Sylvie. *I promised you, and I will try
to keep my promise, though I do not understand you. I will hope
that you change your mind.*

But if Sylvie did not change her mind, Evie thought, staring
out the window into the darkness, could she keep her promise? Could she live in this world knowing that, somewhere, her
nephew was growing up, believing himself without anyone in
the world who cared for him? She raised her head; from the
building across the street came the sounds of an argument, a
muffled shout, a woman's high-pitched protest. She moved to
the window. The woman's shrieks continued, a stream of abuse.
Neighbors began to shout for quiet. She saw a man's head
emerge from a window below, saw a length of white curtain
flutter out beside him into the air. "Pipe down up there!" he
yelled. "Get a divorce already, why don't you?"

A policeman strolled past. Evie saw him glance up toward
the lit windows.

"Now you've woken up Brother Flaherty. He'll call Mayor
Kelly on you." The man in the undershirt twisted in the small
opening between the sash and the sill to pitch his voice at the
open window of his quarreling neighbors upstairs, meanwhile
giving the man on the street below a comic salute. "Good
evening, brother!"

The policeman grinned, tipped his hat. The woman's voice
had quieted now. Evie saw the man disappear inside his window again, though the curtain remained outside, hanging limply
now against the brick wall. She saw the policeman move off
down the street, swinging his stick, his feet making a rhythmic
slap-slap. From somewhere came the sound of music, Louis

Armstrong playing Hoagy Carmichael's "Stardust." The bells at the Ascension Church on the corner struck a single chime— 1:00 A.M.

Evie turned away from the window. She gathered her shoes in one hand and stood beside the bed for a moment, looking down at Sylvie's face. Once, when she and Sylvie were children, Sylvie had been caught lying about failing to pay a visit to an ailing neighbor to whom she'd been sent to bring a box of eggs and a cake. Sylvie had eaten the cake herself with a friend; the eggs they had thrown into the stream, a shocking waste. Sylvie had been beaten with a belt by their father and had fallen asleep finally that night after hours of weeping in bed beside Evie. For a long time, Sylvie's face remained red and swollen. But as the night wore on, Evie saw its expression transform from wretchedness to peacefulness. She had been astounded at the transformation. If she had been Sylvie, she would never have forgotten such shame, even in sleep. But now, her husband dead barely twenty-four hours, her first child lost in the world, Sylvie's face was making itself ready for the next chapter of her life. In the morning, Evie knew, Sylvie would feel better and would feel restless, too—and oppressed by the fact of Jack's burial. Sylvie could be done with sadness quicker than anyone Evie knew. She would not go looking for her baby.

I promised, Evie thought. *I promised.*

Early the same morning, Dr. Hoffman awoke out of a restless sleep. He reached over and picked up the small clock by his bed, but he could not read the hands in the dark without his glasses. He walked across the cool tile floor, carrying the clock to the window, meanwhile unfolding his glasses. Three in the morning. Returning to the bed, he set the clock down on the small nightstand, took off his glasses again, and sat down. He'd been up late, worried about a baby who had run a fever late in the afternoon. By the time Dr. Hoffman had finally left the nursery, just after midnight, the fever had subsided, but he hadn't liked the look of the baby: it lay in the incubator without moving except to protest a little— its mouth moving silently, opening and shutting like a beak —when it was picked up.

On the nightstand was a letter from the incubator manufacturer. He picked it up now to read it but laid it in his lap and sat quietly, instead, thinking. For some time he'd been worried about the filtering system for air blown into the incubators. The cabinets of the incubators were ventilated by fresh air blown through large pipes by fans mounted on the outside of the building. A layer of absorbent wool suspended over a pan of water beneath the incubator served to moisten the air, which was then passed over the surface of hot-water coils and on into the incubator chamber. Though this system was thought to be a improvement over previous models, Dr. Hoffman had felt doubtful about the wool's efficacy as a filter and for some time had been consulting with the Berlin manufacturer about alternatives. Given what took place out there on the streets— and he shuddered to remember the murder of the young man the night before—he was concerned about contaminants unchecked by the present filter system reaching the infants.

He set the letter aside and stood up again. On his reading chair by the window was the hatbox, which he had placed there the night before. He picked it up now, turning it in his hands, running his palms along the smooth sides. It could not have been a coincidence—the boy, the unfortunate boy, was exactly as Alice had described him. You would not mistake that hair, he thought, nor the scar on his jaw. So the boy had brought his baby to the fair in a hatbox, and then he had gone to see the fan dancer. It was certainly hard to account for such behavior. He opened the hatbox again and sniffed inside—the bright scent of a baby's urine.

He would have to tell Alice of the boy's death, that he believed it was the hatbox baby's father who had been killed, though how one explained such a thing he was not sure. All day they had been so busy with the feverish baby that he had not found the time or place to mention it.

Some instinct told him to keep the hatbox, though, and so he put it on the top shelf of the wardrobe and found clean clothes for himself. Thanks again to Dr. Ludwig—he gave a silent nod to his friend. Dr. Ludwig had arranged to have a laundress stop by every other day for Dr. Hoffman's soiled clothes.

What he would have done without Dr. Ludwig he did not know. Dr. Ludwig was well respected in the medical establishment. His affection and esteem for Dr. Hoffman had done much to protect the younger doctor's name, for there were many who would have otherwise called him a charlatan. Yet how could Dr. Hoffman explain now to any of them—even Dr. Ludwig—that he might have chosen differently if he had known, back when it all began, that he would end up like this? Somehow, he'd imagined, there would have been more stability, especially for the Infantorium on Coney Island; as it was, he knew he provided more advanced medical care for premature infants than almost anyone in the United States, and his records—of almost fifteen years now—were invaluable. But he looked desperate, he thought; and in a way he was beginning to feel desperate. Sooner or later, people's taste for seeing the babies would wane; there were already some signs of it on Coney Island. There had been grumblings of disapproval from various morality leagues in St. Louis at the last fair. And other practitioners in Europe, including several who Dr. Hoffman judged had no business in the medical profession in the first place, said their business was just about dried up. There had been letters in the newspapers objecting to his work, to the *Kinderbrutanstalts*—child hatcheries—he organized for the fairs. He had refused to answer such letters in print, feeling it would demean him to do so, but Dr. Ludwig had disagreed.

"It's almost always better, especially in a case like yours," he'd advised Dr. Hoffman, "to appeal to people's sense of charity, to recognize their better instincts."

"Even if they don't possess them?" Dr. Hoffman had asked.

"Even if they don't possess them," Dr. Ludwig had said.

They had been sitting in Dr. Hoffman's walled garden, the night the exhibit in Chicago had opened. Dr. Hoffman was feeling anxious about the day's proceedings, and exhausted, as usual, from trying to oversee too much. Dr. Ludwig's cook had brought them a supper of cold chicken and tomato aspic, a box of white rolls, and a chocolate pie. Dr. Ludwig himself had brought a bottle of white wine.

After several minutes of thoughtful silence between the two, Dr. Ludwig had pulled his napkin from his collar, laid it beside his plate, and leaned over to refill his friend's wineglass. "You look tired," he commented.

Dr. Hoffman smiled, acknowledging as much.

"You know, you don't have to do this forever," Dr. Ludwig said then. He held up a hand as Dr. Hoffman turned to him with an aggrieved face. "No, no. Don't start in on me. I would be the first person to give you credit for your work, you know that. You have done more for the field than anyone else I know. I am indebted to you. And you have meanwhile taught the general public more about common hygiene and infant care than a battalion of nurses could have done. But you *could* close up shop, Leo. You could. You could have a position—on my staff, for instance. But practically anyone would hire you. You could continue your research, without all this"—Dr. Ludwig waved his hand—"fuss."

Dr. Hoffman had said nothing, leaning over, hunched around his glass. What Dr. Ludwig said was true. But he did not want to stop, he realized. Not yet. He wanted to outlast all their predictions, to acquire even more knowledge and skill, to save even smaller babies. Sometimes he was ashamed of his own ambition. It was as if a double rose up in him, a man bolder but less considering, and drove out his habitual caution. Dr. Hoffman could acknowledge this strange twin to himself; in part he could credit it with his success. But he struggled with its presence inside him all the same. Prudence it did not possess, and Dr. Hoffman thought he could sometimes sense this familiar stranger's hectic approach. This other self liked to appear, Dr. Hoffman knew, when some challenge presented itself. Not the challenge of ordinary work—that Dr. Hoffman managed unaided, he thought wryly. But he could sense the division in himself, its approach, in a nearly bodily way: his sleep would grow disturbed, his manner distracted and even haughty, his mind whirring with thoughts almost too rapid in their succession to be apprehended. And he did not know if he trusted this bolder self. Its decisions—quicker, more instinctive— might not always be best in the long run.

He had tried to listen to his own conscience. Was Dr. Ludwig criticizing him? He'd glanced over at him; Dr. Ludwig, whose girth had expanded over the years, was calmly helping himself to another slice of chocolate pie. No, not criticizing, Dr. Hoffman decided. He was being considerate. So in light of Dr. Ludwig's concern he'd thought instead of what lay ahead of him this summer—all these babies. The endless procession of people who would parade through his spotless nursery, expecting to be both awed and reassured, a combination Dr. Hoffman privately thought impossible to satisfy. He himself did not speak during the public tours; often he was too busy, working in a back room concealed from the public. But sometimes he liked to stand off to the side and watch Alice or Nan or one of the other nurses as they made the presentation that he had carefully scripted. He liked to watch the expressions on people's faces when they first came into the cloisterlike room and noticed its cleanliness, its quiet, and its order, the rows of polished incubators and peaceful babies. The spectators looked awed, like pilgrims coming before a shrine, and he experienced a surge of pride so extreme that he sometimes had to turn away to hide his pleasure. He did not like this pridefulness in himself, yet he felt he deserved to be confident about his work; and if the only ones to appreciate him, right now, were these poor people, many so ignorant they had no knowledge of even simple preventive health measures, then he was happy to call himself their teacher.

So he was not ready to give it up; or he hadn't been two weeks ago. But tonight he felt rattled. He might as well just go back to work, even if it was the middle of the night.

It was the boy's death, he thought, knotting his tie slowly and fetching his glasses again from the table by the bed. The boy's death, and the terrible fact that his child, for surely there was no mistaking the connection, was now deprived of a father. It felt to Dr. Hoffman as though something unreliable had been unleashed—babies arrived in hatboxes, young men were murdered on the street. All of it, the entire fair, hundreds of acres of it built on fill, separated from the mainland by the twin bulges of the lagoon—it was all preposterous. Why shouldn't strange forces be at work here?

Even now, the fair's model coal mine, produced almost to scale, was disgorging its rotating load of flashing minerals; prehistoric beasts were shifting and growling in the Sinclair grotto; Madame Zenda, who stayed awake all night to watch the stars for signs of change, foretold the future for a sleepless midget; and a black U.S. Navy submarine rose silently in the darkness from the depths of Lake Michigan. Dr. Hoffman had to reach out to steady himself for a moment against the disorientation that swept over him. He looked down at his hands; what had ever made him think, he wondered in surprise, that he was capable of altering the destined course of a single life? What were his skills against the tidal force of a fate that licked now at his boots? It took all his resolve, a frightening instant of his strength pitted against an enemy he could not recognize— nor, he suspected, did this enemy recognize him—for Dr. Hoffman to continue on his way toward the nursery.

Eight hours later, a little after eleven in the morning, Alice brought him a cup of coffee where he sat at his desk, writing in his notes that the baby known as César Paolo Fluvio, Twin B, the weaker of a pair of twenty-seven-week-gestation twins born to Rosa and Paolo Fluvio on June 4, had succumbed at five that morning, June 10, 1933, of sepsis.

Alice, whose eyes were red from crying and lack of sleep, laid a hand on his shoulder briefly after setting the cup down at his elbow, but he took no notice of her, writing steadily in his small, cramped handwriting with its leftward-sloping letters. After a moment, when Dr. Hoffman failed to acknowledge her, Alice withdrew her hand and left him.

"Causes of morbidity," he began. When he finished writing, he removed his glasses. Some of the nurses had wanted to cancel public tours for the day, but Dr. Hoffman, who had seen the baby moved to the back room, where he and Alice could attend to it, had forbidden this. He did not explain himself to the nurses, but he suspected they took his meaning all the same. *We do not want to convey the wrong impression,* he wanted to protest to Nan Silverman, who brought the nurses' appeal to him and stood waiting while he thought, pulling at his mustache. *Tell them this is a place of life, not death.*

But he said none of this to her. "I think we will proceed as usual, Nan," he told her, handing her his gown.

He added a few items to his notes now: speculations about where the infection might have originated, questions for the medical examiner who would perform an autopsy (with the parents' permission—so few said yes, but it was always worth asking). And then he removed his glasses once again, sat back in the chair, and took a sip of the coffee Alice had brought him, by now cooled to an unpleasant temperature. When he had come into the nursery earlier in the middle of the night, the resident Dr. Sandor and Nan Silverman had just finished rounds, and César's condition—his temperature had returned and was climbing steadily, an unexpected seizure just before three in the morning—had worried the doctor enough that he had been about to come and rouse Dr. Hoffman himself. Together they examined the baby, Dr. Hoffman with a sinking feeling. If it was as he feared, there were so few things that could be done—camphor in oil hypodermically, aromatic spirit of ammonia by mouth. He tried everything he knew; Dr. Ludwig had been called, though he had no good advice, either. As the night wore on and the sun came up and César's condition worsened—he had three prolonged, successive seizures

just after eight o'clock, a dozen apnea episodes—Dr. Hoffman
began to count the minutes.

When the baby died, he was holding it in his arms close to
his chest, standing by the small window in the back room,
looking out over the rooftops of the Streets of Paris.

Alice, who had finally reached the baby's father an hour before, knocked on the door while Dr. Hoffman was standing
there, registering once again for himself the profound and utter
stillness of a dead body—even so small a body as César's.
He'd once expected the weight of a dead baby to change in his
arms, growing either lighter, absent the departing soul, or
heavier, with the weight of death itself. But it always stayed the
same, entirely and forever the same, the clock ticking on,
minute after minute. That was the great mystery of death, he
thought, the shock of it fresh each time. It was the *absence of
change*, what Shakespeare called the "sensible warm motion"
of the body, stilled forever, that took his breath away now.

"Dr. Hoffman," Alice began, "Mr. Fluvio is here . . ."

Dr. Hoffman did not say anything at first. A brown-and-
gray-mottled seagull, its wings cocked, blew suddenly backward past the window over the rooftops in the stiff wind that
had begun earlier that morning, the threshold of a storm that
would at last break the unnatural heat of the past week. Dr.
Hoffman could sense an urgency beginning in him. Though he
did not want to be influenced by such irrational fears, the
baby's death felt like an omen.

He could focus, at least, on César's twin, who, though
stronger from the beginning, might yet be harboring the same
infection that had taken his brother. They were only six days
old, Dr. Hoffman thought, counting back. Six days. And what
had César's life been worth? There was no way to assess the
nature of César's experience. The babies felt pain, certainly;

he had no doubt of that. So, four days of pain and struggle: that's what César's tour in the world amounted to.

Yesterday, Dr. Hoffman thought, he had believed they would all survive; he had willed them to survive. Today he had been surprised by the irrelevance of that belief. Once he had been certain of the force of his conviction, but now he was worried—as much about himself, he realized, as about his patients. Because if conviction counted for nothing, if babies still died, even if you swore they would not, then conviction was pointless. You were only standing on water, pretending it was solid ground.

Dr. Hoffman looked down at the tiny, swaddled form in his arms—César's blue mouth, lips compressed. Little gums arrested. Empty mouth. Little lashless eyelids pressed closed.

"Dr. Hoffman?" Alice was waiting at the door. "Leo? Mr. Fluvio—"

"He is too late," he said finally. "I am afraid he is too late."

He was persuaded to go and sleep for a while by Nan Silverman, who finally sent him and Alice away to rest shortly after one that afternoon. They had all agreed that César's body should be transported to the funeral home in the incubator ambulance, rather than by hearse, so as not to excite suspicion in the crowds of fairgoers.

Dr. Hoffman had found himself almost speechless before the Fluvios. He suspected they took his manner as respectful, and it was, he thought, though he'd wished he could say something more, say anything, as he saw them out the door, Rosa Fluvio supported on her husband's arm as he helped her down the steps. Watching them, he found himself wondering—for the first time; that's what troubled him now— what it would be like to have a child of his own. To have a child, and then to lose it.

He walked back into the nursery; the noon showing had just finished. Dr. Hoffman surveyed the room; all seemed in order. But there was no one with the hatbox baby. Dr. Hoffman crossed the room and stood before the baby's incubator. The child's color had improved, but he thought he detected a tightening in the facial muscles, the suggestion of effort. He had pleaded with this baby not to die, but that wish, he saw now, had been more selfish than anything: *Don't die; I'll look a failure.*

He frowned, leaning forward, and put his hand to the glass wall of the incubator. *I cannot even begin to imagine what you are going through,* he thought. *And you cannot tell me, except by the mute and terrible distress of your body.*

He felt suddenly exhausted. Across the room, he saw the white backs of his nurses, babies in their laps, swaying in the rocking chairs, their white feet planted, two by two, on the black tile floor. Someone's foot was tapping—a rhythm steady and slow, the labor of the heart and lungs. He looked back at the hatbox baby. He bent nearer. At the infant's temple, the blood under the skin rose and fell, rose and fell; the nurses rocked; the foot tapped. His put his finger involuntarily to his wrist, felt his own pulse slow to match the percussion that now filled the room, the frail sound of endurance.

SEVEN

It was early, a little before six, when St. Louis left the lagoon at last and headed toward the Lido. The air was still cool; the streets were clean. A breeze blew in from over the lake. Behind the clouds, the sky was lit with a demon red that augured a storm.

St. Louis crossed the street and headed through the empty turnstiles at the gates to the Streets of Paris. The entrance building to this section of the fair was modeled to look like a huge landlocked steamship cresting onto the fairgrounds from between enormous metal waves painted in bold shades of turquoise and amber. Visitors passed from America to France through the belly of this ship, beneath two squat funnels tilting jauntily toward the stern.

"Here's where you'll get your *real French atmosphere!*" the barkers called all day. "Cafés, bars, artists' quarters, dancing, music, no cover charge!"

St. Louis looked up and sniffed the air as he pushed through the turnstile. He'd be glad of rain. It might wash away his own growing sense of turpitude and regret.

Six sleepy-looking waiters, their damp hair combed slick and brilliant, their aprons stuffed in their pockets, and their shirt collars unbuttoned, sauntered along the sidewalk ahead of him toward the Café de la Paix and the Café de la Rotonde in a cloud of aftershave. A heavyset midget woman, her arms crooked upward like a hat rack, her black hair in two huge rollers, waddled past him on the other side of the street, string bags of groceries — bulging oranges and glinting cans of coffee — swinging from her biceps.

At the Lido, St. Louis climbed the steps and let himself in with his key. Inside, he headed down the dark hallway, past a dozen red plush chairs haphazardly stacked along the wall, toward the back of the theater, where the dressing rooms were located.

He knocked on the door of Caro's dressing room and sniffed; someone inside was smoking. Walking back from the lagoon, his mind full of the baby in the hatbox and Hoffman and his own uncertain future, he'd decided he needed some honest task to perform, something that was not too complicated but would make him feel occupied and productive. Doing his washing was just the thing. The laundress came twice a week, but he'd always liked washing clothes himself.

He hadn't counted on Caro's being in her dressing room that early in the morning, though, much less smoking. He'd thought she'd be asleep still, either in her private apartment around the corner, on the second floor over a women's shoe store, or in the hotel she sometimes escaped to on Michigan Avenue.

"It's me," he said, leaning toward the crack of the door.

There was no answer. St. Louis frowned, turned over one hand, and examined his fingernails, waiting.

"I know you're in there, Caro," he said after a minute. "I can smell smoke."

From inside the room, he heard the creak of bedsprings and then the sound of Caro's feet crossing the floor. He stepped back as he heard the lock turn in the latch.

But the person who opened the door wasn't Caro. It was Sullivan, the big Negro who worked with St. Louis sometimes as Caro's bouncer. The rest of the time he worked maintenance on the rides at the midway. He was agile and quick, despite his formidable size; he was one of the men who climbed the Ferris wheel to make repairs.

"Well, you don't look like a fan dancer," St. Louis said.

Sullivan grunted and returned to the bed where he had been lying on his back, smoking a cigarette and reading St. Louis's copy of *A Tale of Two Cities*. Caro's ostrich-feather fans were crossed one over the other and hung on the wall across from the bed. But her clothes were strewn everywhere: over the floor, across the backs of chairs, and in heaps on her dressing room table.

"Where's the early bird herself?" St. Louis asked over his shoulder, walking around the room and picking up Caro's clothes from the floor.

"Out." Sullivan didn't look up from the page.

St. Louis straightened up with a pair of panties in his hand and shook them at Sullivan. "Now tell me the truth, Sully. Who are you hiding from this time?"

Sullivan looked over the top of the book at St. Louis. "She's a *nice* lady. She offered me a place to nap because I didn't have no *sleep* last night. Said she was going out for a walk."

That wasn't like Caro. Neither the early rising nor the walk-

ing. St. Louis bent over and picked up a blouse, a pair of stockings, Caro's robe, which had been crumpled up into a ball.
"How come you didn't get any sleep?"

Sullivan only grunted again. But then he laid the book face-
down on his chest and looked up at St. Louis. "I spent my
night being charitable and mopping up a man's blood what got
spilled all over the street. And then I was so sick I went and
had some beer with them Indians, and then I was too awake
and rattled to sleep. I'm trying right now to settle my *mind*."

Sullivan picked up the book again as though he were going
to take up where he'd left off, and then he set it back down over
his chest. He rolled over onto his side, closing his eyes. "You
usually the busiest body around, St. Louis. Where you *been*?
Didn't you hear a man got murdered last night?"

St. Louis turned slowly and stared at Sullivan.

Once, as a child, St. Louis had sat almost without moving for
a whole afternoon, waiting a long time in a dark hallway until a
door had cracked open at the end, admitting the mournful, wet
green light of a late-summer afternoon. The hallway had been in
his aunt and uncle's house, and he had waited there for news,
just as he waited now. That day, so long ago, he had held still in
a long agony of anticipation; and once, in a moment of everlasting strangeness, he had felt himself divide into two—the self
who waited, and the self who watched him wait. He had seen
himself leave his own body, take a few steps away down the
hall, and then turn around to frown at the little figure of stone
who remained behind, sitting cross-legged and unyielding on
the stair landing. It had been long, long ago, the light of the disappearing day outside moving across the wall, a searchlight
proceeding down the hall, picture by picture, as the sun ranged
across the sky and prepared to set. Eventually, the doctor had
come out of Caro's childhood bedroom, holding his black bag.

St. Louis saw again the faded blue wallpaper of the hall, the gray scene of an unfolding cataract surmounted by an arched Oriental bridge. An avalanche of rounded boulders and carefully etched ferns rolled away into the nothingness of the wallpaper's blurry background. St. Louis had looked up when the door opened, and it had felt strange to move, for he'd sat in a trance since after lunch and now it was almost suppertime. The doctor had not seen him at first but had stood by the door a moment, slowly unhooking the stethoscope from around his neck and folding the rubber tubes in his fist. When he glanced up at last and found St. Louis waiting there, a small figure at the end of the hallway, he had smiled. He came down the hall, and when he drew near to St. Louis, he came down to one knee.

"Go on and pick your cousin some of those pretty posies I saw out there in your aunt's garden," he said to the boy. St. Louis had watched the doctor's experienced eyes flicker over his face and body, taking measurements, assessing the bulging brow, the stocky chest, the short legs. But the old man had only smiled, patting him on the shoulder. "That'd be a gentlemanly thing to do."

The doctor's visit had been the beginning of St. Louis's first separation from Caro; she'd had scarlet fever, and St. Louis had been banished finally to a neighbor's home until Caro recovered and the house had been scalded and scrubbed. St. Louis remembered now the sensation of waiting to have his worst fears confirmed. It had lasted for weeks. Every day, he had set himself a new test of endurance, holding his breath underwater at the lake, or climbing one branch higher in the magnolia tree, or doing cartwheels down the stairs. They were feats of audacity he offered up to the gods—*watch me risk my neck*—to bring her back. But he also understood them as an exercise in readiness, preparation for a lifetime.

Every day, he jumped into the haymow in the neighbor's barn from one rung higher on the ladder.

Every day, until the reports started to sound promising at last, he was ready for someone to come and tell him Caro was dead.

Sullivan sat up again, a cigarette in his mouth, looking for a light. St. Louis stepped forward with a match. Sullivan's head, the hair shaved so close to the skin you could see the blue-black color of his scalp, was huge, an effigy's; his palms flashed white around the flame St. Louis held out toward him. "Some man nobody knew got killed by some man nobody knew," he said, and St. Louis shivered. Sullivan hunched his shoulders once, quickly, as if a fly had landed on his neck. He rubbed the fingers of one hand together and looked up at St. Louis. "Poof. Up in smoke. They're both gone."

St. Louis stood still, trying to piece together what he had heard with what he had both seen and sensed last night: Hoffman sitting on the curb, the hatbox beside him. The strange feeling in the street, that something evil had walked down the center of the road, scattering ordinary citizens. The aura of violence he had felt. Now he knew something solid, though the knowledge sickened him—a man had been killed . . . , and somehow the hatbox, and presumably its contents, had been orphaned in the wake of that accident. A wave of cold ran over him.

"And nobody saw *nothin'*, neither," Sullivan said. "Just a plain meanness murder. You know." He made a motion like plunging a knife. He took a drag of the cigarette, looked down at it in his fingers. "Guy killed wasn't even more than a kid, practically."

St. Louis almost didn't want to ask, but he'd come this far. Shouldn't he know the rest? "What did he look like?"

Sullivan looked up at him incredulously. "You think I took a *long* look? You think maybe I wanted to remember that my whole life?" He shook his head. "You something, St. Louis. It was a kid, I told you. Redheaded boy. Skinny."

St. Louis took a breath. A door slammed somewhere, far away in the recesses of the Lido—the wind, maybe, blowing through the double doors that led from the alley into the dark orchestra pit.

It was confirmation, but confirmation that came with the impact of a blow. That redheaded boy with the hatbox.

But the baby—what had happened to the baby? And did Hoffman have him now? And why on earth would someone have killed that frightened-looking boy?

"He didn't have a . . . a baby with him, did he?"

Sullivan gave him another look, this time of disgust. "A *baby?* What are you *talking* about, St. Louis?"

"Forget it." St. Louis glanced around the little room—signs of Caro's habitual untidiness everywhere, pots of makeup uncapped on the dressing table, clothes and books and newspapers and cups on the floor. There was nothing more to be learned here. He stuffed the last few things on the floor into the laundry bag.

"I'm sorry, Sully. You're a good man."

Sullivan raised a palm in farewell but did not open his eyes.

"Sweet dreams." St. Louis closed the door behind him.

The cord of the laundry sack bit into St. Louis's shoulder as he walked down the street. He passed the Café de la Paix: Three filthy gulls gripped the iron railing, rocking back and forth; one opened a beak wide as St. Louis passed, but no sound came from its throat, which worked up and down, up and down, as if trying to disgorge something vile. A woman's single shoe, black, with a pearl button, lay on its side under a café table, the heel snapped. Shards of a broken glass flashed in the gutter. A white cloth napkin was tied inexplicably around a chair leg, securing it to the railing.

St. Louis turned the corner. The storks at the baby house had climbed to the rise of the small, bare mound overlooking their fountain and pond. They stood utterly still, their white feathers almost transparent in the thin morning light. They were turned toward Lake Michigan and the sky, where fists of black clouds were gathered now near the horizon.

As he passed the incubator exhibit, St. Louis realized that he was expecting Hoffman in some way, expecting him to come out onto the steps and lift a hand toward him, a gesture of their complicity. For if Hoffman indeed had the baby, it was St. Louis who had, in a way, delivered him to Hoffman's door.

He stopped a moment, staring at the closed doors. He and Hoffman had been brought into range of each other now, as unlikely as that seemed. The possibility of Hoffman and St. Louis having anything to do with each other was unthinkable under almost any circumstance, St. Louis recognized. But the way Hoffman had sat there on the curb last night, his whole attitude of being *unprepared*—St. Louis could not understand that. He himself always had something ready, something up his sleeve. He had learned that one should always have cigars or cash to dispense, jokes to tell, or lies; trick locks that sprang open in your fingers, or stacked decks of cards, or wooden nickels. He was surprised to find himself thinking of the doctor, of this man who cared for the most fragile of human beings, as unequipped—even, he thought, in some vague danger.

And then it happened again, just as it had happened that day so long ago when he'd sat waiting for the doctor to come out of Caro's room. Then he had stepped away and looked back on himself, he recognized now, with pity, his whole, small world hanging in the balance while Caro hovered between life and death. Now, for a moment, it was happening again: He could leave himself on the street and trespass into Hoffman's rarefied world, where one man took over the unfinished work of so many women's wombs. In one fleet, stealthy motion, St. Louis could pass through the walls of the hospital and come to Hoffman's side in the nursery filled with the forced sound of artificial breath.

But St. Louis had to stop there. Because if he put out his hand toward Hoffman—a gesture of comfort, or only the wondering touch of one creature trying to recognize another—it would pass through Hoffman's body and into the immaculate air beyond. He could stand right next to Hoffman and breathe into his ear, and the doctor would never hear a sound.

A guard at the art museum let St. Louis use the laundry facilities in the basement of the museum in exchange for tickets to Caro's show or, if St. Louis was out of tickets, the chance to hold one of Caro's undergarments for a few minutes.

"That's enough," St. Louis would say, snatching Caro's brassiere from the old man's fingers after five minutes. "Ante up, Dad, if you want more time."

Sometimes, grumbling and complaining, the old man would rummage in his pockets for more coins (though St. Louis usually found a way to return them, unnoticed, to the baggy pockets of the guard's jacket). Lenny was thin as a whippet, his gray hair combed neatly; the teeth marks of the comb left a visible trail over his skull. He had shaking hands— from a slowly worsening palsy—a loose-lipped mouth, and a rubbery face the color of steak, which he could screw up into comic expressions.

St. Louis liked him. The man had a terrible lovesickness for
Caro, but he'd never in a million years approach her, let alone
harm her. He told St. Louis he'd been married once, to a funny
woman with double-jointed knees, but his wife had left him so
long ago that he hardly remembered what she looked like, only
the image of her bent backward over the bed, laughing and
laughing, her legs folded up strangely beneath her. He didn't
do anything dirty with Caro's clothes. He just sat there and
held them, like a man holding a baby. He thought Caro was a
goddess.

"How come she never got married?" he'd asked the first
time St. Louis had shown up with a sack full of dirty clothes—
he and Lenny had first become acquainted over the card table
at the Café de la Paix. Lenny had led the way down to the museum's endless, echoing basement, his heavy jailer's ring of
keys clanking against his narrow thigh. "Wait, I know, I know"
—he'd held up his hand in the dim stairwell as if to silence
St. Louis, descending the steps behind him. "There wasn't one
good enough. Am I right? I'm right. Who could be good enough?
Who could lie down next to that every night and not have a
heart attack? I'd have a heart attack." He shook his head,
unlocked a door. "It's better I just sit in the back row."

In the basement, St. Louis had pulled the chain. A cone of
white light—the light of the interrogator—fell over them
both. The walls were lined with caged enclosures containing
crates and oddly wrapped shapes. Two industrial washing ma-
chines were set up in the center of one area; two long metal tables were set end to end over a floor drain.

"What do they wash in here?" St. Louis had asked Lenny
out of curiosity, loading his shirts and trousers and Caro's silky
underclothes into the tub.

"Huh?" Lenny had looked up at St. Louis; he'd been mesmerized by the appearance of Caro's clothes. He cupped a hand around his ear.

St. Louis sat down on a crate and lit a cigar.

"No smoking," Lenny had said sternly, gesturing at the cigar. He folded his arms. "You want to know what they wash? I'll tell you." He came over and sat down next to St. Louis, crossed his legs. "Mummies." Lenny cackled.

St. Louis had smiled and taken a playful poke in Lenny's direction. There were three mummies in the museum, loaned by the Egyptian Museum in Cairo. They were small things, St. Louis had noted, looking at them in their dimly lit glass cases; they were *his* size, actually.

Lenny had grinned, happy. "Seriously! You ever smelled a mummy? Close up?" He'd turned aside discreetly and held his finger to his nose.

This morning, though, St. Louis was in no mood for Lenny's banter. He'd found him dozing lightly in front of the old masters. The old man jerked awake when St. Louis touched his shoulder. A group of people, including a pair of twin boys in sailor suits, holding their mother's hands, and a group of older women with name tags pinned to their flowered dresses, were filing through the room, silent and expressionless, past Tintoretto's gushing *Venus and Mars, with Three Graces in Landscape,* past Bartolommeo Veneto's *Portrait of a Youth,* past Piero di Cosimo's *A Lady Holding a Rabbit.*

Lenny opened his eyes and smiled at St. Louis, then reached up his hands to St. Louis's shoulders and patted them.

"Hi, Dad," St. Louis whispered, leaning down. "Got something for you."

Usually St. Louis didn't mind satisfying Lenny's harmless wish to hold something of Caro's in his hands—he never went off to the men's room and did anything dirty to them, after all.

He was just a lonely old man. But today, the whole business seemed pathetic to him. In the basement, he rummaged through the sack of dirty clothes, extracting socks and shirts, blouses. Lenny stood a pace or two away from him, waiting quietly. As if sensing St. Louis's irritation this morning, he looked pointedly away from the proceedings, as if he had nothing to do with them.

St. Louis pulled Caro's dressing gown from the bag and shook it out. He turned around with an attempt at a flourish—there was no need to make Lenny feel bad, he thought; let the guy have his fun—but when the robe unfolded stiffly in front of them, covered with dried blood, Lenny stepped backward, his hand over his heart. "Jesus!"

St. Louis almost dropped the dressing gown. The blood had dried in waterfall patterns all down the front of the robe and had drenched the hem.

Lenny's face was white.

"Don't have a heart attack on me now." St. Louis hastily put the bathrobe back in the sack, found a cup on the edge of the deep metal sink, filled it with water, and stood over Lenny while he drank it down, his hand shaking.

"What happened to my girl?" Lenny said. "Jesus! Is she all right, St. Louis? Tell me she's all right. Nobody tried to hurt her, huh?"

St. Louis pulled out a chair and sat down. "Sully saw her this morning. She's fine." But the sight had shocked him, too. Somehow Caro must have been there last night, had been present when that man—*could* it really have been the baby's father, that *kid?*—was killed. What had happened to bring her anywhere near that scene? It almost looked as if she had sat down in the street in a puddle of blood. "You okay?" he asked Lenny.

Lenny waved a hand at him. "Gave me a shock, that's all."

St. Louis saw that Lenny was embarrassed now by how emotional he had become. He leaned over and picked up the laundry sack. "You go on back to work. If you can call it work, sleeping in front of art." He smiled, trying to cheer Lenny up.

Lenny stood shakily. "Okay," he said. "Okay, St. Louis. I'll be seeing you."

Lenny put both hands on the banister as he began to climb, and it was that gesture, the gesture of an old man hauling himself up the dark stairs, hand over hand, that made St. Louis rise to his feet in a burst of impotent anger. There wasn't anything he could do for Lenny except bring him this poor substitute for affection and relief—the ghost of Caro's presence. He couldn't do anything for the hatbox baby, or the baby's father, or . . . and where was Caro herself? What questions could she answer? It would be like her to be elusive right now, just when he needed something from her.

But what was it he needed? he thought, leaving the museum. He needed information, first—he *must* be right about the baby's father. Sully had said the man who died was nothing more than a boy, and redheaded—all that would describe the young man St. Louis had seen, the one he'd led to the doors of Hoffman's hospital. And there was no mistaking that the young man's hatbox had been the same one Hoffman had carried away with him on the street last night. But where was the baby now? That was the question.

Where was that boy's little baby?

He hurried toward the Lido, through crowds suddenly so thick that they appeared to have grown magically from between the stones of the streets while St. Louis had been in the museum, human beings pulled vertically from the underground and set to walking, their faces flushed, their eyes restless, their hands clutching. Despite its nights of abundant stars, despite its entertainments and diversions, despite the distracting wands of color that crossed over the lagoon at sunset like beams from a sorcerer's wand, despite the magic and the miracles and the money, all that *money*—you could *hear* it falling into vendors' boxes, chink, chink, chink—this summer had felt to him like a slowly narrowing tunnel.

He'd been fighting the sensation for weeks now, the sense that one morning he would wake up to find a cold stone wall close before his face, all his chances for escape sealed over. He wanted a reason to leave now that would be finally more powerful than his devotion to Caro, the force that had kept him by her all these years. Was there anything stronger than that? What was stronger than love? he thought.

But he was afraid to answer that question.

The news of the murder should have made him feel especially determined to move on, he considered, passing the gates of the Nocturnal Gardens of Enchantment. During the day, without the lurid light show, the gardens looked like an ordinary public park, neatly edged paths, displays of flowers, trees pruned into sculptural shapes. And yet the murder was creating in him instead a fresh and urgent sense of purpose: to see things through, somehow, before he left. Though what that would mean, or how he would ever manage to leave Caro, or what he would do if he did, he couldn't have said.

This whole fair is about the future, he thought, *about what we can see ahead, what we think the world will look like tomorrow or next week or next year or even in the next century.* And yet he could not see beyond his own two hands stretched out before him. For the first time in his life—and here he was, *surrounded* by the future, an explicit future, artfully envisioned— he found that he could not imagine what would come next.

His favorite souvenir from the fair so far was a little cardboard box, not much bigger than a deck of cards, with nine little windows in it. Behind each window was a bit of some material—a chip of sillimanite or iron ore or zinc, a tiny nest of mohair, a pinch of cotton, a bit of cork, rubber, glass, asbestos. MAN MUST GO TO THE EARTH FOR ALL MINERALS, read the lettering over the top of the box. St. Louis had figured out how to remove the face of the box so he could take out each item and touch it. He thought it was funny that the fair—this fair, where everything was turned into something else, where the invisible energy of electricity filled the air, where everything moved by unseen forces, where everything was shown and yet nothing was revealed—should be promoting something so plain and elemental as this collection of ordinary artifacts.

But he treasured the little box and its contents. He liked to be reminded that everything had its source in something plain and solid to the touch. Glass, for instance—even a whole house made of glass, even a world made of glass, he thought— was nothing but silica sand, soda ash, limestone, and salt.

Caro had come back to her dressing room once but had gone out again, Sully reported to St. Louis when he returned to the Lido.

And she was not in the Café de la Paix, where she sometimes liked to sit alone and do a crossword puzzle and eat lunch, protected by a phalanx of waiters. St. Louis supposed she had gone into the city to shop, but he was annoyed by her disappearance, and vaguely worried. He went to the afternoon showing at the baby house, but Hoffman was nowhere in sight, and a new nurse, one St. Louis did not recognize, was giving the talk. It distressed him that he could not figure out which baby might be the baby from the hatbox. He stared at the row of incubators, the swaddled infants inside them, their faces tiny and indistinct. And then it occurred to him, for the first time, that maybe the baby hadn't lived.

Suddenly he wanted to get outside.

When the rain started at last a few minutes later, after having threatened all day, he found he had no energy to move. He stayed where he was, watching people scatter into cafés and shops. Steam began to rise from the ground; those pedestrians who were left hurried through the downpour on invisible feet, black umbrellas tilting above them. The 250-foot Ferris wheel on the midway slowed to a standstill; the last of the passengers, disgorged from cars the size of school buses and equipped with red plush seats, were deposited safely on the ground, where they ran for cover, programs and newspapers folded over their heads. Flags and pennants clung wetly to the poles. Across the fairgrounds, the colored electric lights of the buildings blazed through the rain—the Rainbow City, they called this fair— but because there were few windows, another nod to economic necessity, the landscape now looked eerily uninhabited. An insubstantial ballet of watery light played over the buildings, giant hunks of stone and steel that appeared to have collapsed and fallen into decrepitude like a lost civilization. Discordant strains of music—the thudding of Indian drums, the patriotic shrill of tin whistles, the melodies of waltzes—slowly ceased as musicians took their instruments indoors. The air was instead full of the whispering hush of steadily falling rain, the press of Lake Michigan's waters rocking against the shore, the screeching cry of a gull that sailed alone down the center of the street, trailing the distant odor of the sea.

St. Louis was still sitting on the steps of the baby house when the afternoon showing let out; people came down the steps and divided around him like floodwaters around a tree. One woman with a little boy drew the child away from St. Louis sharply as he stood up, soaked to the skin. A light rain still fell. He turned away, knowing that his condition at that moment—wet through, his hair plastered to his misshapen head—would frighten her. But he was not fast enough, or maybe his own haste had alarmed her, and he heard the sharp intake of her breath, saw her stumble as she tried to hurry away. The little boy looked back over his shoulder as he was dragged off, and St. Louis saw the frank curiosity of his gaze. The child had been to see every manner of strange thing on earth, all there to stand up and be gawked at; what would be the difference to him now, staring at St. Louis?

St. Louis had nowhere to go except his stifling room in the Lido. He walked down the street, the rain falling around him. At the Café de la Paix, the glass doors that protected diners from bad weather had been pulled across the terraces, and the green canvas awnings, opened and unfurled. The glass had steamed up inside. St. Louis could make out only the indistinct blur of people leaning toward one another over the tables inside, someone's red jacket, a waiter's white back, the dark cap of a head. A low hum—intent and conspiring—met him on the street.

At the museum, his feet leaving a trail of wet footprints, he found Lenny. Sympathetic, silent, Lenny led him with a hand on his shoulder to a distant chamber, a small hallway between two empty galleries. It contained only a single piece of sculpture, the head of a Greek warrior mounted on a black pedestal, the pugilist's nose chipped, his eyes empty, a lock of hair curling over his beautiful forehead. A low leather settee was set before a Palladian window overlooking the rain falling out on Lake Michigan, the gray sky. St. Louis lay down as Lenny pressed his shoulders back against the cushion.

His last sight before he fell asleep were the sails of a three-masted schooner, Byrd's South Pole ship, a thing from the past fighting through the rain at the dim line of the horizon, disappearing into the clouds.

EIGHT

Sent away by Nan Silverman to rest after the Fluvios had left the nursery, Dr. Hoffman surprised himself by eventually falling into a deep sleep that lasted nearly six hours, the longest stretch he'd had in weeks. When he awoke, the sun was just beginning to set, and he found himself hurrying as he showered and dressed.

When he lifted his chin to knot his tie, he knocked his glasses off; they dropped into the sink under the mirror, where one of the lenses fell out. He had been away from the nursery for too long, he thought, sitting down at the table and putting the broken glasses in front of him on the blotter, trying to arrange the lens into the eyepiece. He shouldn't have slept that long. He couldn't see very well for such close work without the glasses; it was a maddening business, trying to repair them. Finally, after several minutes, the lens was in place again. He fitted the glasses over his eyes and blinked. He cursed his poor eyesight as he hurried down the hall. He had lost precious minutes.

In the nursery, a group of wet nurses were beginning the

first evening feeding. They looked up as he came into the room; conversation between them halted. Dr. Hoffman hesitated a moment but then only nodded in their direction and went to wash and put on a clean coat.

When he came back into the main room, though, he decided to stop and speak to them. He should greet them, say something cordial and friendly. No doubt they had been disturbed by little César's death; he should reassure them that all was well.

He wished he himself could feel that all was well; his eyes still ached, as though he hadn't slept at all. He resisted the urge to rub them.

There was no reason to take the baby's death harder than any other, he told himself. Still, it was a disappointment.

"I see you are taking good care of our little Helen." He stopped before one of the girls; he wished he could remember her name. He could always remember the babies' names, but the wet nurses' identities swam in his mind. He let Alice tend to them mostly, after his initial lecture, usually delivered from behind his desk, about strict cleanliness, about the importance of their diets, about keeping their own infants out of the nursery.

The girl smiled down at the baby at her breast. "She's such a tiny little thing. She don't take much. Not like Joe." Her eyes fluttered up toward Dr. Hoffman's face and then quickly away. "Joe's my boy," she said.

Dr. Hoffman began to pull at his mustache and then put his hand away, into the pocket of his jacket. From across the room, he saw Alice glance in his direction. The girl pushed off with her foot, sent the rocker moving at a gentle pace.

Dr. Hoffman cleared his throat. "She is stronger already, though, than when she came, no?"

"Oh, yes! Much! I see the difference." Her expression was surprised, as if Dr. Hoffman had guessed the correct answer to a difficult question.

He found himself interested in the girl's certainty. He did not usually ask the wet nurses for their opinions. Alice conveyed to him anything she thought he would find significant. "How so?"

The girl blushed. "I couldn't say."

"No, go on. Please."

The girl looked down at the baby in her arms. It was almost lost in the plump fold of her elbow. "Well . . . " She hesitated. "It's how her eyes are."

Dr. Hoffman frowned. "Her eyes?"

The girl looked worried. "Not her eyes, exactly. I mean . . . how she feels." A pained look came over her face; pink flooded under the surface of her skin. The baby dropped away from the nipple, its mouth open, a drop of milk on its face. It looked half-dead.

The girl bent over her quickly, touched the baby's cheek with a finger, coaxed it toward the breast again. "There's my girl," she murmured, her lips close to the child's head. "There's a girl."

Dr. Hoffman stood there. He looked away toward Alice, but her eyes were on him, and he shifted away from her gaze. He did not know if he should extricate himself from this conversation.

"I mean—" the girl began again suddenly, surprising him, "I mean, she knows what she's about more. She knows *me*."

Dr. Hoffman moved back a step, away from the rocker's inching progress toward his foot. He felt suddenly in the way. He was not used to feeling in the way in his own nursery.

"Alice—I mean, Miss Vernon—she says that's a good thing,"

the girl continued quickly. "When they know you, they've taken a step forward." She looked up at him for confirmation.

"A step forward—" Dr. Hoffman tried to steer his mind toward what she meant, toward the significance of this.

But the girl sat up straighter in the chair, suddenly confident. The baby had fallen from the nipple again and lay back against the girl's rosy arm. "All right now," the girl said cheerfully. "Don't wear yourself out. Tomorrow's another day." She lifted the baby to her shoulder. One hand came up and cupped the back of the infant's tiny head. It vanished entirely behind the girl's white palm. Dr. Hoffman found himself suddenly imagining the softness of the girl's pillowy breast, the excellence of a woman's body . . .

"You have . . . everything you need?" He could not think of what else to say, but he felt suddenly grateful to her.

"Oh, yes," she said. "Yes, sir." But she was not looking at him. Her eyes were half-closed, her cheek tilted toward the baby's head. "I'm good at this."

It wasn't an answer to his question, exactly, but he thought he could make the leap that took her from what she needed to her sense of purpose in the world. A fragrance came from them, the woman and the baby; yet Dr. Hoffman could not exactly place it.

"You are very . . . necessary," he said urgently. "Very necessary."

The girl sent the rocker going again.

Dr. Hoffman hesitated. He leaned toward her. She seemed almost asleep. "I'm sorry, your name . . ." he said finally. "I'm afraid I have forgotten . . ."

Her lashes opened. She smiled up at him from her drowse. "It's Frances," she said. "Frances Martin."

"Yes." Dr. Hoffman felt obscurely relieved. That *was* it. He *did* remember now.

"Dr. Hoffman?" She had raised her eyes again, though she held one hand still between the baby and Dr. Hoffman. He could not see the infant at all; it was cocooned in Frances's breast, the blanket draped over them both.

"I'm sorry about little César," she said. "We're praying for his brother."

He found himself reddening. "Thank you."

And then he turned away. Alice was crossing the room, holding out a baby toward him. The telephone began to ring. One of the babies began to cry, a little cry, unutterably sad.

He felt ashamed as he walked toward Alice. He had thought to reassure the girl, Frances. But she had comforted him, instead.

He stayed at the nursery until after ten that night, when Dr. Ludwig dropped by unexpectedly and insisted on taking him out for a late dinner at Wilson's Roof Garden Restaurant. The rain had finally stopped. A waiter mopped off their chairs before they sat; puddles had collected on the seats.

They were served steaks on sizzling platters, rolls with butter, salads.

"I'm sorry about the baby." Dr. Ludwig poured wine for them.

They talked about the nursery for a while, about the possibility of the infection that had taken César spreading to the others; of course Dr. Hoffman had taken measures against this, isolating the remaining twin. Though only time would tell, of course. They could only hope, really.

But Dr. Hoffman could sense that his colleague was distracted. He knew Dr. Ludwig was a sympathetic man; the deaths of his babies wounded him. But his somberness this evening somehow did not seem connected to César's death, and Dr. Hoffman's inability to assess Dr. Ludwig's silent mood only made Dr. Hoffman more anxious than he had been all day — and the day before, too, he thought. Ever since presiding over that awful death in the street.

He pulled irritably at his mustache and made some notes in his pocket notebook about questions he wanted to ask the oxygen supplier.

Finally he pushed his plate away.

After dinner, Dr. Ludwig ordered a bourbon with a dash of bitters and a lump of sugar. Dr. Hoffman waved away a drink and sat quietly, his hands folded on the tablecloth, looking out over the twinkling fairgrounds. Rainbows of colored light wavered in the humid night air. People moved below them under the artificial lights from the streetlamps, a mass of heads. Dr. Hoffman sniffed. He could smell peanuts. Below, he watched as the organ-grinder and his white-faced monkey, Capuchin, with their paper sacks of salted peanuts, crept slowly around the corner with their cart and took up a position near the restaurant. Dr. Hoffman, who was fond of peanuts — good source of protein — had exchanged pleasantries with the organ-grinder; all his years on Coney Island had given him a sense of comfort with street people. Many were from eastern Europe, and sometimes they would speak German or French or Italian together.

"I am afraid I have rather unsettling news," Dr. Ludwig said suddenly. "I have been thinking how best to tell you."

Dr. Hoffman turned to look at him.

"There will be some letters in the Sunday papers." Dr. Ludwig lifted his glass, sighed, took a sip of his drink. He did not meet Dr. Hoffman's eyes. "Apparently, there is some . . . moral opposition to the exhibit."

Dr. Hoffman groaned. He covered his eyes with his hands and pushed the heels of his palms across his forehead. "I wish you wouldn't call it that," he began. "You know I hate the term. It's really not—"

"I use the term only for expediency." Dr. Ludwig leaned forward, held Dr. Hoffman's eyes. "Dr. Hoffman, I must tell you. The person organizing the campaign against you is . . . a woman." He sighed. "She is, in fact, the wife of one of the trustees of the fair. He has been to see me; it is, of course, a rather awkward position for him. I am afraid he feels helpless to dissuade his wife. She is—they are—extremely powerful people."

"What are you suggesting?" Dr. Hoffman looked away from Dr. Ludwig, down at the street again. A cluster of men in polka-dot clown suits, their red noses shining, blundered wildly through the crowd below, jostling people. He saw passersby turn in annoyance. *They're drunk*, he thought.

"I would like to propose a meeting," Dr. Ludwig began. "An invitation, in fact, so that you might—"

"Certainly not. No." Dr. Hoffman frowned. He watched the clowns disappear around the corner. He began, almost as if he had rehearsed this speech, "I will not defend myself or my work to—"

"You may not have a choice," Dr. Ludwig said quietly. He finished his drink, put the empty glass down on the table, and pushed it away with a finger.

"What do you mean?"

"Only that, as I said, these are extremely powerful people. I think your best hope is to try and show them what you do, the good of your work, the sincerity of your medical practices. You can do that with ease. I will do what I can, of course, and I have already arranged—"

"I don't want you to do anything." Dr. Hoffman spoke abruptly.

Dr. Ludwig sat quietly. Together they looked out across the fair. The lighted Sky Ride cable car moved slowly over the lagoon like a spaceship. Dr. Hoffman thought uneasily of all the people poised there up in the air. Clusters of green and gold and pink fireworks went up in a bright spray over the lake. The two of them watched the sparks fall toward the water.

"You see," Dr. Ludwig said finally, turning back to Dr. Hoffman, "I am afraid that because of this lady's . . . associations, there is very little that can be done. Should she gain sufficient publicity and support for her efforts, and I am sorry, but I must tell you, as well, that her sister is married to the paper's editor"—Dr. Ludwig grimaced apologetically at Dr. Hoffman—"there is little question in my mind that the nursery will be closed before the end of the summer."

Dr. Hoffman sat silently. He should have been prepared for this, he thought. He had been prepared for it, some day perhaps. And yet it didn't seem exactly real, Dr. Ludwig's warning. He felt extraordinarily tired. For a moment, the baby César's face flashed before him, the infant turned to stone, just like the stone children in the public garden fountains of his youth. The only child of two cultured and preoccupied academics, Dr. Hoffman had spent much of his childhood alone, without the company of other children, tended to by a series of nurses and tutors. His imagination had been seeded and had taken root in that isolation. Sometimes he thought he would never get over the habit of being alone. How did one do it? How did people move so apparently effortlessly into the stream of life, traveling down one branch and then another?

"What exactly is her objection?" he asked finally. But before Dr. Ludwig could answer, he went on hurriedly. "And aren't we making too much money for the fair, in any case? They would not want to—"

Dr. Ludwig interrupted him. "You can imagine the nature of her objections," he said, "even though they are based in ignorance. You have heard such things before: that the babies are treated like animals or freaks, that it is a crime of human decency to parade helpless children before the public in such a way. You know all this, what people say. But it is less important what she thinks. I can tell you that the board will close you down rather than suffer an onslaught in the papers—and she is connected enough to organize an onslaught—regardless of how much money they stand to lose. They see bad publicity as more costly, in the end." He leaned forward. "That is why I think your only choice is—"

"All right." Dr. Hoffman put up a hand. "I understand what you are saying to me. You are telling me I need to fight."

"Not fight." Dr. Ludwig smiled. "You are too good for a fight." He looked fondly at Dr. Hoffman. "I'm sorry," he went on. "I did not predict this, and I would not have invited you to come here this summer if I had suspected such an outcome. If the complaints were coming from anywhere else I would agree with you that perhaps it would be best to ignore them, though I've always thought you could protect yourself better by being forthright about your work." He waved away an approaching waiter. "Tell them of the difficulties of funding research in your field! Show them the results of your years of work! Produce incubator babies grown up into sturdy young men and women, happy children saved from death!" He sighed, picked up his empty glass, looked at it critically. "But I am afraid this is a foe that cannot be brushed aside easily."

Dr. Hoffman sat quietly; his stomach was upset. Either way, he thought, his reputation was at risk now—whether he chose to court his opposition or ignore it. He could not close down the nursery without appearing to have conceded some irregularity

—the novelty, at least—of his position. And yet to engage in his own defense was equally humiliating.

"I have asked Mr. and Mrs. Taft to dine with me," Dr. Ludwig said, "on Saturday night."

Dr. Hoffman looked over at him.

"There will be time, you see, for Mrs. Taft to retract her letters, if you—"

"If I am sufficiently . . . persuasive," Dr. Hoffman said.

Dr. Ludwig smiled. "Exactly."

Dr. Hoffman and Dr. Ludwig parted company on the street.

"Remember," Dr. Ludwig said. "Come at seven. Black tie." He put a hand on Dr. Hoffman's arm. "Perhaps all will yet be well," he said. "I have always rather wanted to see you test your charms with women, anyway," he added, teasing. "I think they may be considerable." He smiled.

"I do not think that testing my charms, as you call them, with someone else's ignorant, hostile wife, is where I ought to begin," Dr. Hoffman said. "But I'll be there."

He watched Dr. Ludwig walk away. Dr. Ludwig was a handsome man, tall and weighty, with finely shaped, almost feminine eyes and a high, clear forehead emerging from a receding hairline. You could see his intelligence in his face. Like Dr. Hoffman, he, too, was unmarried still, but he had a longtime mistress whom Dr. Hoffman had met on one of his trips to Chicago last year, when the nursery was being planned. She was half-French, independent minded, vivacious and lovely, and possessed of a not inconsiderable inheritance with which she bought art, though Dr. Hoffman, whose tastes were entirely conservative, could see little value in her selections of abstract paintings. Still, her affection for Dr. Ludwig was obvious, and he had felt jealous of Dr. Ludwig. Most of the women Dr. Hoffman seemed to encounter were poor or downright destitute; most of them were the mothers of the infants in his hospital. He simply never met suitable companions.

He had planned to return to the nursery briefly before retiring for the night, but he wasn't sleepy and found himself walking instead, turning over in his mind everything Dr. Ludwig had said. As he walked, the streets gradually emptied around him. A mist began to fall, not so heavy as to dissuade him from his walk but dispiriting enough that people were going home early. Soon the streets were empty.

He walked down the abandoned main avenue of the fair, passing the shallow black waters of the lagoon on his left and Lake Michigan on his right, toward the Adler Planetarium, whose domed glass roof glowed ahead in the misty darkness with a greenish light. The planetarium formed the outermost anchor of the fair, surrounded on three sides by Lake Michigan and linked to the fairgrounds by the strip of bathing beach and the agricultural buildings, which now, in the wet air, sent forth the smells of the animals housed there, the cows and sheep, horses and goats. Dr. Hoffman registered the odors; they were earthy and welcome, reminding him of his grandparents' summer farm in the Netherlands, the low white buildings there with their view of the sea, the slow-moving herds of sheep that drifted over the hills. He had been happy in that place.

A generously proportioned walkway planted with pleasant shade trees ringed the circumference of the planetarium building. During the day, people liked to pause here beneath the fluttering leaves and watch the white sails of boats on the lake, the regattas and pleasure craft. Dr. Hoffman reached the planetarium and stopped at the railing to lean over and look out at the dark water below him. Tonight, the lake's vast indifference

set up a yearning in him, making him think not forward into
the future but back in time, assess his choices and decisions,
relive with a sharp and sudden regret all the ways in which his
life might have been different. For a moment he felt tempted
just to give up, give in, let this Mrs. Taft have her ignorant way.
He could, as Dr. Ludwig had suggested many times, simply
join Dr. Ludwig's staff at Sarah Morris. He could buy a house,
find a wife . . . and yet why did this seem such an illusion to
him, this prospect of normalcy?

He did not think he could bear to work for someone else,
even someone as admirable as Dr. Ludwig. He needed to have
things done in his own way, to let his instincts for medicine
have free rein. Those instincts, he knew, more than anything
else—more, even, than his years of training—made him a
good doctor. Sometimes, he saw a baby as a kind of playing
field, saw its future marked out as a course that wove between
opponents and risks. He had to be free to *imagine* what would
happen, a calculated series of moves that would dodge and
evade disaster. Every time he saw one of his graduates—some
were now young men and women and came back to visit the
Coney Island hospital with their parents, producing their nursery baby bracelets to prove to him who they were—he felt vic-
torious and marveled at the way they walked or spoke, the way
they wore their hair, how they held themselves.

Was this, too, a dangerous feeling? he wondered now.
Should he not simply have gotten to his knees in the face of
every living child, thanking God instead?

He left the water's edge finally and drifted toward the shadowy agricultural buildings, thinking. The barns and pavilions
were open to the night air; tied-back tent flaps twitched in the
wind, tugging against their ropes. He had never been in this
part of the fairgrounds before; the familiarity of the animal

smells surprised and pleased him. As he passed the entrance
to one barn, he saw at the far end, positioned before an open
door that looked out toward the lake, a ring of men sitting motionless on crates around the circle of light thrown from a lantern on a small table. The men's backs were rounded over
hands of cards. They did not look up as he passed. The grass
and straw underfoot made his tread noiseless.

He walked through one barn, invited in by the inquiring
face of a horse, thrust suddenly over a stall door toward him.
He stopped to hold the creature's nose in his hand, feel its
warm breath, and then walked on, past the quiet, heavy bodies
of the sleeping cows, their heads dropped low, toward the dim
light at the end of the barn. Here the grass gave way abruptly
to a rocky ledge; beyond was the bathing beach and the smell
of the water.

Though it was hard to see in the dark, he found a way down
to the shoreline through the rocks. He stood for a moment in
the cooling sand at the bottom. Above and behind him he
could see the dim lights of the fair; yet it seemed so far away,
so quiet, down here by the water. His mood—what was it?
Why did his heart beat so fast? He had started walking to rid
himself of worry, he thought, to steady his mind.

The babies. All the babies. He had never weakened before
in the face of his responsibilities. The challenge of setting up
the nurseries, of managing the finances, not to mention the
medicine—these had exhilarated him. And yet now he felt
himself failing the babies in some important way.

How would the Fluvios mark little César's death? he found
himself wondering. What was there to be said about such a
brief life? He realized he had never been to a service held for
an infant he had lost. Had he been asked and refused to go? Or
did the families see him as culpable in some way? He would

be the man at the back of the church, no seat saved for him, the congregation turning at his approach. Had Alice ever been? What did the grieving families *do?* he thought in bewilderment.

Put my baby in a paper boat and sail it off to sea—where did those words come from? A bit of a song he'd heard. He turned toward the water, looked out into the dark. Now, coming toward him in a flotilla of tiny paper boats lit with candles, would be all the babies he had lost. He was astonished to realize he could remember each one of them—there had been fifty-two in the years he'd been in practice in the United States, sometimes several in a cluster if some infection passed through a group, and he saw them come before him now, a moment from each child's brief life, sometimes only its last moment, the infant held in his arms or Alice's or, more rarely, its own mother's. How strange: he could even remember the time of day each child had died—those near dawn, those as the sun set, those who went away at noon and never came back. He remembered them all.

He was so sorry, he thought now, about César. So very sorry.

He stood there, the imagined line of departed infants in their dream boats sailing away again after giving him their benediction, the little lights of their lives dimming. And then he registered first the sound of distant splashing and then the sight of someone moving through the water ahead of him, swimming perhaps twenty feet from shore. He took a step closer to the water's edge. The swimmer moved past swiftly, plying the water with steady strokes. At the jetty at the end of the bathing beach, the figure approached the shore and emerged.

It was a woman.

Dr. Hoffman fumbled for his glasses, but in a moment they were misted over and he had to take them off again. The woman—he could see her figure well enough, though not her face—leaned over to pull on a pair of trousers; he saw her heavy breasts fall forward, her long limb raised to slip into the trouser leg. By the time she had pulled on a shirt, she had already begun walking. Dr. Hoffman could see that she held a pair of shoes in one hand. She disappeared over the far side of the jetty.

Dr. Hoffman followed her at a soft run over the sand, then through the dark and shadowy and abandoned fairgrounds, watching her as she moved from darkness into light and then back to darkness again beneath the streetlights. All right, she was a vision, he thought. But she had swum out of that other vision of a circle of babies in their paper boats, his own personal catalog of loss. She had reached the end of someplace in the company of those children. And then she had returned— returned to him—breaking the invisible barrier between death and life.

He kept his distance behind her; in one part of his mind he felt appalled at what he was doing.

But he had recognized her now, and he could not lose her. He did not think he could bear to lose her.

She walked along the shore of the lagoon, parallel to the lake, vanishing in the curtains of the willows' lacy branches and then reappearing for a tantalizing moment before vanishing again.

And then he realized she knew she was being followed.

He stopped, alert, humiliated; what did he think he was doing? But he began to walk again, quickly now, because even worse than the prospect of being discovered by her was the prospect of failing to catch up with her, take her by the arm, turn her toward him so that he could look into her face and be certain. He had seen her just that once, when she knelt over the dying boy in the street with him; but he realized he had been holding the memory of her there inside him, a thing just out of range of his recognized thoughts, a kind of wild, unlikely alternative to everything that seemed to be happening to him. *There* was desire, he thought. *There* is what he had been missing.

Now she had disappeared into the concealing skirt of a tree, only to double back somehow, perplexing him, to be closer than she had been before. It happened once, twice. He stopped again, his breath coming fast, his face flushed. If a gun had gone off somewhere in the distance, he would have fallen to the street.

And then, just before the bridge that spanned the center of the lagoon, she was there, standing on the path in the darkness before him.

"You're the doctor." He could not see her face, but he thought she was smiling, the way her voice sounded. "Do you always follow women about at night?"

"Of course not." He stopped several feet away from her, held up his hand awkwardly—*I won't come any nearer*. "I'm sorry."

Yet he was so glad to see her; he had not expected to be so glad. What had he thought after that night they had knelt over the boy dying in the street? That she would appear just that once, a literal angel of mercy, and then vanish. For he could not go see her, he could not visit the fan dancer in her rooms, nor watch her dance while he sat shoulder to shoulder with so many other men. It was impossible, anything between them— the fan dancer and the doctor.

But now, here she was: she had come out of the waves, out of the water—how astonishing!—swimming toward him. He was so happy—the idea almost struck him as funny, and he began to smile—he was so happy that he thought he had never been this happy before in his life. Never. This is what she did to him.

No wonder they paid money to see her. He looked at her under the trees, the lamplight falling around her; her hair, wet and dark, was the color of plums. She was so beautiful.

"Of course not," he said again, embarrassed and yet pleased.

And then he bowed, a gesture from his boyhood—he had been taught to bow to ladies, though no one, certainly not in America, did such things anymore.

The next night, as he was dressing for his dinner with Dr. Ludwig and the Tafts and whomever else Dr. Ludwig had thought to invite who might be helpful to their cause, as he was knotting his bow tie and inspecting himself in the mirror, he thought that what had happened, the baby doctor and the fan dancer together in one of the Ferris wheel's swinging cars, high up in the night sky during a storm, was an example of life's rarest and most wonderful ironies. It was, he thought, not the sort of thing that happened to him at all. And yet it had.

He had bowed to her as they stood there on the path by the lagoon, and when he had stood upright again, a huge black man had appeared beside her.

"Sully," she had said, "meet Dr. Hoffman." So she had known his name, too.

Had this man been with her the whole time, watching her swim and then watching Dr. Hoffman follow her, keeping his own stealthy distance until Caroline turned to face Dr. Hoffman on the path? Was this man her bodyguard?

"Sully, could we go up there?" She had turned away from Dr. Hoffman, her bemused inspection of him, and pointed up to the sky.

He had not understood her meaning at all at first—what was she proposing? It almost seemed she meant *flying*, that she was asking this huge black man whether she and Dr.

Hoffman could be endowed with the gift of flight for the night, and that this Sully was capable of granting such wishes. Dr. Hoffman had felt reckless: Of course! Flying! He would do anything.

But she had only meant the Ferris wheel. Sully had helped her into one of the enclosed cars and followed Dr. Hoffman in safely with his eyes, and then a moment later the wheel had started with a lurch, and they had risen high up above the fairgrounds into the night sky. Dr. Hoffman had caught at the bar on the seat before him. Caroline had laughed and put her hands next to his, and he had laughed, too.

It had been like being in a boat up there, the darkness all around them, sailing in the wind and the rain, which began again after a few minutes. Dull, soft, shuddering flashes of distant lightning broke somewhere over the flat, soaked fields of Illinois, illuminating her face near his own as they sat side by side on one of the bench seats, holding on to the silver bar before them.

She had wanted to know more about the boy in the street. What had happened? What did he know?

He had taken a deep breath and then told her everything. About the coincidence of it, the terrible coincidence of it. About the baby in the hatbox—the tiny infant so surprisingly steady and strong. He had told her about César Fluvio. He had talked for—how long? Hours, it seemed. She had asked a few questions, and he had from time to time paused in the stream of his descriptions to take in the sight and smell of her close beside him.

At last he had stopped talking. "You must think I'm mad," he said at last, "talking like this. I don't know why . . ."

She had smiled, and he thought in shame that perhaps men always did such things with her, always found themselves hell-bent on confiding something, as if her companionship had to be earned through a river of confession. Or maybe it was just a way to keep her here next to him: *Talk fast enough, and she won't be able to get up and leave.*

"It's all right," she said. "It was interesting."

He had turned to her beside him. They sank into the horizon of the fair again and then lifted free of it, the car swinging gently. Every time they neared the ground, he grew anxious. Every time they rose in the air, his heart rose, too. He could feel her next to him, her thigh against his. She smelled of the lake water—like a water nymph, he thought, and enjoyed the fancifulness of the notion.

"I've always loved fairs," she said, leaning forward and putting her chin on her hands, looking out over the lights.

"Have you?"

"It was so boring, where I came from. It was a farm. I thought the sameness of it would kill me."

"You like . . . something new. Every day." He smiled at her.

"Oh, not every day."

He waited.

"I like to be surprised," she said finally. "I'm continually amazed, now."

He thought that he, too, courted change, courted the unexpected. Why else work in this profession? Dr. Ludwig called it a—what? A frontier. All medicine was a frontier, perhaps.

"You, too," she said, as if she had read his thoughts. "You could have been something boring."

He shook his head and laughed. "You are right. The babies are never the same. Every one is different."

"But . . . you must have children of your own?"

"No," he said, surprised. "No, I have no children." She had sounded so certain; he realized that perhaps it was odd—this man who spent his life holding babies in his arms had never held one of his own. He hadn't ever really thought about wanting children. Now, suddenly, the desire for it rose up in him— it was as if she had put something foreign and delicious to his lips and let him have a taste.

"And you?"

She looked at him and then gave a short laugh. "Me? No, I'm afraid not." She laughed again, but he saw that he had embarrassed her in some way.

"And you are not . . . married?" He wanted to be sure of this.

She turned to look at him. For a long moment she examined his face.

"I only ask . . ." He jumped in before she could answer. "I only ask because . . ." And then he reached over and put his hands on either side of her face and held it. "Because one day I would like to see the man who has found perfect happiness."

She smiled at him, but he could feel the smile, too, her cheeks lifting under his fingers.

"When I was a little boy," he said, "my mother and I would play a game at night when I was going to sleep. It was called 'the perfect day.' We would say everything we could think of that would make a perfect day." He smiled at her. "Mine always ended with éclairs."

She reached up then and put her hands to his face, holding him just as he held her. "And your mother?"

He had to think now, reeling at Caroline's touch. What had his mother wanted? "It would end like this," she had always said. "Here with you." And he had heard a wistfulness in her voice. He stroked Caroline's hair. "She was like you," he said instead. "She wanted something new, every day."

Caroline leaned close, put her forehead against his. "The perfect day. It doesn't exist."

"Oh yes, it does," he said. "Because I'm having it."

And then he kissed her.

She had stood up at last and leaned across him to the little window beside his seat. "Sully!" she called. "We'll come down now."

The car had lurched, and Hoffman had felt the descent in the pit of his stomach. He'd wanted to make love to her.

"I have a dinner engagement tomorrow," he said hurriedly. "But I will be back at the hospital—I have rooms there—after eleven or so. Would you come? Come and have a glass of wine with me?"

She sat back down beside him, took his hand.

"There's a walled garden, my private garden," he went on. "There's a door in the wall. You could knock there, anytime."

Dr. Hoffman saw the fair's dark horizon swing up suddenly before him, the flat line of the world tilting, the buildings pale gray and soft and shadowy. The colored lights had been switched off. The sun had not risen yet, but a thin, clear line of dawn showed at the edge of the sky.

"Won't you be tired?"

"No!" he said. But she was smiling at him. "All right. Yes. Yes, I will probably be tired." He leaned forward and kissed her again. He wanted to take her shirt off, wanted to put his hands everywhere on her body. "But I won't feel it if I know you will be coming. And then when you do come, I will be fully awake. That I can promise you." He bent his head, kissed her neck. *My God. She is so sweet-tasting.*

"All right," she said. "I'll try."

They had stepped from the car. Sully had been nowhere to be seen, but Caroline had turned and given Dr. Hoffman her hand.

"You are not what I expected," he said to her, and then regretted it when he saw her eyebrows go up.

He bowed his head and brought her hand, enclosed in his own, to his burning forehead; he squeezed her hand, closed his eyes. "I meant—"

But she was smiling. "Good night, Dr. Hoffman," she said. And then she walked away, hurrying along the path by the lagoon.

In a minute, he could not see her anymore.

That night, as he was dressing for dinner with Dr. Ludwig and the Tafts, he stared at himself in the mirror one last time, giving his tie a final adjustment, before leaving his rooms and going to face his enemies. *It doesn't matter anymore what happens to me,* he thought, *as long as I have her near me.*

He checked himself now, staring at his own face in the mirror. *Do I really believe that?* he wondered.

But all around him, as he climbed into the car and gave the driver sent by Dr. Ludwig the address of the restaurant, all around him as they drove toward the city through the fairgrounds, was the image of the future, the unimaginable given shape and texture and weight and presence. He almost wanted to reach forward and stop the driver, to get out and walk, to feel himself part of the crowds that moved through the loveliest hour of the day in this place that had suddenly become, for him, the source of Caroline's pleasure—something new, every day.

Wait, he wanted to say. *Stop.*

But the car was moving forward. If they did not hurry now, he would be late.

NINE

A day later, a few minutes before Caro's first show of the day on Monday, St. Louis, wearing one of her silk kimonos over his trousers, stretched out on the daybed in her dressing room, lit a cigar, and opened the Sunday newspaper. Smoke billowed around him. "Listen to this." He waved the cigar in her direction. "'Learn taxidermy,'" he read aloud. "'Have fun! Make good money in your spare time, too.'"

Caro glanced at him from the mirror where she was fixing her hair. "Put that thing out. It stinks."

St. Louis ignored her and read on. "'Learn to mount and preserve all kinds of birds and animals and fish. Tan skins and make them into rugs and robes. Take common specimens like rabbits, squirrels, frogs, et cetera, and make them into ashtrays, mirrors, lamps, *et cetera.*'" St. Louis rolled over on the bed, howling with laughter, bringing the newspaper with him.

Caro stopped brushing her hair and made a face.

"Look." St. Louis struggled to sit upright, still wheezing with laughter, and held out the crumpled newspaper to show her the photograph of a white baby bunny, eleven or so inches tall, standing on its hind legs for all eternity. Held on its stiffly outstretched paws was an ashtray containing a smoldering cigarette.

"Ugh!" Caro turned away in disgust.

St. Louis laughed again, took another puff of his cigar, and then stubbed it out in a tin can filled with pink sand at his feet. "Just what you need in here. A frog ashtray. A bunny ashtray."

"What are you reading those ads for?" Caro tugged at her hair, looking at him through the mirror.

"I need an occupation." He didn't look up from the page. "I need a career. I could do this in my spare time. It says so." She made no reply to this, but he hadn't expected her to. Every time in the past when he'd mentioned striking out on his own, Caro had said nothing at all, neither giving him her blessing nor begging him to stay. "Why don't you get down on your knees?" he'd asked her once, when he'd threatened to stay behind in Coney Island.

"It wouldn't make any difference whether I did or not," she'd said. "You'll do what you want."

"No," he had complained. "That's you. *You* do whatever you want. I just tag along because I have no better alternatives." She had kissed him then, put her cheek briefly to his. "You know I'd be miserable without you. Who'd boss me around?"

Caro began pinning up her hair. St. Louis put down the newspaper and watched her. When he had tracked her down finally Saturday evening after her last show, he had laid out for her the connection he'd made between the murder and the baby presumably delivered to the fair's incubator exhibit. But she'd been without questions about the event, complaining of a headache and saying she wanted to go home and go to bed. He supposed it had shocked her, seeing the boy dying in the street like that. How had he died exactly? Suddenly it seemed important to know that.

"Whatever made you go out there?" he'd asked her.

"I don't know," she'd said. "I just had a bad feeling."

So she had disappeared Saturday night, leaving him alone and with nothing to do except go and wash dishes at the Café de la Paix, where he broke three glasses, cutting open the oyster of flesh at the base of his thumb with a nick that bled profusely. All day Sunday she'd stayed out of sight, too. And though they'd eaten dinner together Sunday evening at the Old Heidelberg Inn on Leif Ericsson Drive — a silent dinner, full of sentences almost begun and then abandoned — when they had finished she had again excused herself early and said she was going home to read.

He'd paid their check and then trailed her reluctantly from the Old Heidelberg, bored and lonely.

"What are you reading these days? *Quo Vadis?*" It was a joke; the only book Caro had read — the only book he'd ever seen her read — was Henryk Sienkiewicz's best-seller about a love affair between a Roman officer and a Christian woman, set in Nero's Rome. The book had been extraordinarily popular. St. Louis, who liked to read and considered public libraries society's most important achievement, had just finished Sinclair Lewis's new novel, *Ann Vickers*. He would have liked to talk to somebody about it.

They'd been standing on the sidewalk outside the restaurant, waiting for the car and driver St. Louis had hired this summer for Caro; Maxfield, as the driver called himself (St. Louis was sure it wasn't his real name) was another of St. Louis's poker friends from the nightly game at the café.

"Don't you ever get tired of old *Quo Vadis?*" he asked again. But then he glanced over at her and saw that, for a minute, she couldn't think of what to say. A funny expression had come over her face, as if she'd been given a gift she already possessed and now had to appear pleased and surprised nonetheless. And then he had known that she wasn't reading anything at all.

"You're the worst liar I ever saw," he'd said in disgust, and had walked away.

"Hey," she called after him. "Don't you want a ride?"

He hadn't turned around. "I don't want to ride with you," he said. "I'm mad at you."

For a minute, Caro didn't say anything. "Suit yourself," she called finally.

If she was sleeping with someone, she ought just to tell him, he thought, marching off down the sidewalk. He hated that she was always so cagey about such matters. For a woman who took off all her clothes and danced in the nude, she was ridiculously private about her sexual affections.

Now Caro put down her brush and came over and sat down on the bed next to him. He scooted over to give her room. She frowned, plucking at his sleeve; the flowers crumpled in her fingertips, contracted, and fell open. "I wish you'd take this off," she said. "You'll ruin it." But she leaned back against his shoulder and looked at the paper with him.

"Hey, look at this." St. Louis sat upright.

He read silently for a moment. "Listen," he said then. "It's a letter to the editor. 'Notwithstanding Dr. Leo Hoffman's credentials, the exhibition of any infant or infants undergoing the process of artificial incubation in any place of amusement or public resort, or in connection with any amusement enterprise, violates our every sense of decency and propriety as human beings. That such unfortunate babes are to be exhibited alongside fat women, catchpenny monstrosities, fire-walkers, and fan dancers should and does offend our deepest sense of integrity and charity. While not accusing either Dr. Hoffman himself or the fair's trustees with cupidity, we strongly encourage Dr. Hoffman to remove his precious and fragile charges to a more proper and suitable environment and leave the public to marvel instead at such worthy exhibits as the glorious Court of States or the Horticulture Building and its charming gardens.'"

St. Louis held the paper out to Caro. "They don't like you, either, obviously," he said. "Think of that—you and the baby doctor, maligned by the same pen."

But Caro only sat quietly beside him, looking away and tugging gently at the tassel on a pillow as if it might pop open and reveal something inside.

"That'll be bad news for the baby doc." St. Louis looked back down at the paper. He didn't know whether Hoffman had ever survived such threats before, but it certainly wasn't the first time someone had taken a shot at Caro. She'd never seemed to mind it much; in fact, she said the assaults—strident, hysterical, pompous—amused her.

He felt the bed move as Caro stood up.

"I need to get dressed," she said. "Go see if Billie and Cass are ready, will you?"

St. Louis looked at her. She had turned back to her dressing table.

"I need to get dressed," she repeated pointlessly.

He made a noise of impatience. "Don't you have anything else to say?" He held the paper toward her, as if to remind her of what it contained. "Aren't you *interested*?"

She shrugged. "In what way?"

St. Louis stared at her. "I don't know," he said. "It just seems like . . ." But he couldn't decide what to say. He got up

after a minute and took off the kimono. He was always struck
by the fact that Caro referred to preparing for her show as getting dressed, when it fact it meant getting undressed. She was
modest around him; she didn't let him stay in the dressing
room while she prepared herself, patting her skin with the
thick court plaster that gave her such a glowing and concealing
uniformity. Of course, he'd seen the show — Caro was very
graceful, and funny, too; that was part of her charm, he thought.
She winked at the audience, smiling with what St. Louis recognized as a kind of winning intelligence, as if she shared the
joke, never once revealing her entire body, only tantalizing
flashes of it. And certainly she was beautiful. This summer
she'd hired two additional dancers, Billie and Cass, sisters
who danced inside ingenious big bubbles and allowed Caro
both to shorten the amount of time she herself was onstage and
to pique the crowd's interest even further.

Caro waited while he put his shirt on.

"You want me to hang around?" he asked. "You want to
have dinner at the café later?"

Caro shook her head. "You don't need to stay. Sully will be
here. He wants the extra money, anyway." She looked away
from St. Louis a moment and then turned to her dressing table
and opened a drawer. "Here," she said, holding out a fifty-
dollar bill. "Don't go picking on any little rabbits."

St. Louis looked at the bill held in her outstretched hand.
For a moment, as it lay there on her palm, St. Louis had a sudden, sickening vision of all the hands it had passed through, all
the ways in which it had been exchanged for objects, services
— a plate of Brunswick stew, a shave, a length of rope, a pedi-
cure, someone's toes under a paring knife. "What are you giving
me money for?" he asked quietly.

She shrugged, but he could see her expression tense.

"I was kidding," she said. "I don't want you scalping any baby rabbits to make an ashtray. I don't want you needing money."

"I *don't* need money. I'm the only guy in America who doesn't need money. You give me plenty of money." He stared at her. He could feel his own expression becoming belligerent. This felt like a bribe of some kind, though for what, he wasn't sure. She was paying him off, but he didn't know what he was supposed to do—or not do—and he didn't like the implication that he could be distracted by a fifty-dollar bill.

"Jesus," he said. "Jesus, Caroline. What is it that you want, anyway?"

She turned around and put the bill away. "Suit yourself," she said, but her tone sounded forced to him, deliberately casual. "You're awfully huffy."

"I don't think it's me who's huffy," he said. "I don't . . ." But he didn't go any further. He stared at Caro's back, the lovely hourglass shape of Caro's back. He'd hit something there— he'd embarrassed her, caught her at something. If she hadn't actually been trying to pay him off—though for what, he couldn't understand—she at least had been trying to get rid of him. That much was clear. But why? For a moment he had a brief image of himself boarding the train, case in hand, and disappearing from Caro's life.

She wouldn't look at him now. He didn't know what was going on, but he didn't want to hurt her. They'd been together too long, he thought. And then a creeping guilt came over him. For the first time, he had not thought that he couldn't bear to leave her, but that she might be wounded if he went.

He had not thought about how much he loved her, how he couldn't do without her.

He had thought the way he supposed a well-intentioned

man or woman in a long, wearying marriage might think—that what held them back from leaving was the sheer accumulation of years, a force of weight so oppressive that it prevented, after a while, even the desire to escape it. There was only the holding still.

He had not thought about loving Caro. For the first time, he had not thought about loving her.

The shock of that realization made him suddenly nervous, as if he had to account for some span of time he could not remember. He glanced around Caro's dressing room. It was pathetic, the way she lived. Even her apartments looked like a place someone stayed in while they were between things. She couldn't cook anything; they always ate out. She didn't really own anything except a lot of clothes, and even these she sometimes just left behind when they moved. They made friends easily enough—people wanted to befriend Caro, of course; who didn't want to be the beautiful fan dancer's friend?—but then they lost them when they left, sometimes never to see them again. Once, when they were in New York one winter and living in a hotel, he'd bought her a kitten, a thin, gray-striped creature, with ribs like delicate ivory stays. She'd adored it, let it rip up a lot of her clothes and the hotel's silk-upholstered chairs, and made a bed for it in her own bed out of a rose-colored cashmere shawl. But when they left, he found out she'd given it to the Irish girl who cleaned their rooms.

It occurred to him now with a sudden shock that she had no permanent address. Neither of them, as long as they'd been together, had had a permanent address. *What a way to live,* he thought. *Why have we been living this way?* Suddenly, the sight of Caro's hands busy with her hair, fumbling with pins, filled him with regret—and a cold embarrassment. It seemed the sun had slipped silently from the universe altogether, an Alaskan winter settling down over them. A fan up at the high window blew a dry breeze down on his head. The tap at the sink in the corner began to drip. When Caro bent to retrieve a single pin that had fallen silently from her hand to the floor, her fingers searching blindly under her chair, he had to leave.

"Forget it," he said now. "I'm sorry."

"OK." She waved vaguely through the mirror but did not meet his eyes.

He wanted to say something to her, something that would restore not just the moment but the past and the future, too. "Caro . . ." he began.

"Break a leg," he said.

Their joke.

And then he shut the door.

He put Caro out of his mind, though the effort felt furtive, more as if he were simply trying to evade her, losing himself in the fair and thereby losing her. That afternoon he went and swam in the mild, murky waters of the lagoon, though people were not supposed to swim there, wading in through the sand and clowning around and floating on his back and sending forth burbling plumes of water from his mouth, pretending to drown and delighting a group of children on the boat dock, until he was told sourly to get out by a policeman. He went over to the fire walkers' exhibit and crashed their show, hopping over the coals, howling and grabbing at his feet, making the onlookers laugh. He took on two of the pirates—fellows he played cards with at night sometimes—at the children's mossy Enchanted Island, knocking them into the water and falling in himself, until people screamed with delight. He danced with the agile and good-natured taxi dancers and mimed a man swooning with love. He stuffed bills into the girls' dresses, sang snatches of song. He sent trays filled with bottles of beer to a group of drunken Swiss tourists sitting with their wives, straw-colored women glistening with sweat and rolled up inside their dresses like fat twists of sausage and lard. He joined a troupe of wandering musicians and persuaded one of them to give up his accordion, and then he swayed down the street making awful noises. People clapped.

And then, exhausted—he had *needed* to be exhausted, he thought, to distract himself from feeling sad—he went to the baby house. He didn't expect to be let in to see the kid's baby—if the baby was even there. Was he supposed to knock at the door? *Excuse me, have you got a baby from a hatbox in there, by any chance? I knew the father* . . . But he wanted to come close, anyway. Maybe he'd see Hoffman, the great doctor, the great man who had sat on the curb the other night, the empty hatbox beside him. What had he been thinking? The astonishing surprise of our lives, the endless, unexpected shock of how we both begin and end? Hoffman—the great doctor, maligned in the newspaper. The great doctor, that miniaturist of medicine, who saved lives. The great doctor—showman, charlatan, overseer, ringmaster, or saint? How could you put all those pictures together?

But the baby house was closed; the last show had finished two hours before. A single couple stood at the fence in the gathering twilight, their two children—with heads of hair so blond-white that they looked, from a distance, like tiny wizards—reaching their arms imploringly through the bars, murmuring, trying to cajole the imperious storks toward them. For a moment he imagined the storks inclining their ugly heads and the children climbing onto the white backs, the storks rising up into the night air, difficult wings slowly beating, the children waving. *Good-bye, good-bye.*

When St. Louis approached, the family moved off quickly, the man herding his children under his arms like ducklings, the little white-blond wizard children tripping under his feet, silent and sleepy.

Then a plump young woman in a flowered blue dress, her eyebrows drawn in heavily with a pencil, her lips smeared pink, came out and sat down on the steps. St. Louis saw her fumble in a white purse and extract a pack of cigarettes, then search for a match.

He moved to stand in front of her. "Light?"

She looked up.

He watched the familiar series of expressions travel over her face—surprise, wariness, and then relief. It was the lack of calculation in his face that relieved people.

He grinned at her and pretended to search his pockets. Failing to find anything, he pulled a perplexed face. "Gosh," he said, patting himself—the top of his head, his knees, his elbows, the flapping soles of his shoes. "Gee. I know I've got 'em somewhere."

She smiled.

He continued to pat his pockets, and then, as if he had suddenly discovered something under his fingertips, he reached out a hand and snapped his fingers. A match sprang to life.

She opened her eyes wide.

"Go on," he said. "It's hot!"

She laughed and leaned forward to light her cigarette.

He wiped his brow. "Whew."

She glanced sideways at him and smiled. "Well, you're not a very experienced magician, are you." She had a funny mouth— with tiny teeth, blunt as corn kernels—that made St. Louis think suddenly of monkeys with their stuffed cheeks.

Her name, he discovered, was Louise. She was one of the fif-

teen wet nurses working for Hoffman and Alice Vernon at the
fair that summer. ("It's all right," she said, shrugging. "We get
plenty to eat, anyway.") Her own baby boy—Tiger, she called
him—was eight months old. She was not married. Her parents
knew Dr. Hoffman from Coney Island, where her mother was
the cook at the Infantorium on the weekends, providing steaming plates (plain white china, blue rim) of breakfast, lunch,
and dinner for Hoffman and the nurses; she brought home left-
overs sometimes—spiced beef falling from the bone, chicken
paprikash, ham and beans. Her father repaired shoes and always smelled of leather. She loved Charles Laughton. She'd
seen Katharine Hepburn in the movie *Morning Glory* three
times. She liked walking around the fair, sitting at the Café de
la Paix and drinking a coffee (milk, three teaspoons of sugar—
Dr. Hoffman let them have one cup of coffee a day). She and
the other wet nurses would watch one another's babies while
they looked around the fairgrounds like regular tourists.
Sometimes one of the other girls would come with her at night
and take a walk, but tonight they were playing cards. She didn't
like cards. She never won anything and it was boring. She was
nineteen. She was five foot three and weighed 151 pounds—not
in her shoes. She wanted to work in a department store, selling
gloves and hats, or jewelry. She had pretty hands, good for
showing off rings—see? Her birthstone was emerald. She
hoped to be wildly rich one day. Did he know J. P. Morgan had
paid $51 million in income tax between 1917 and 1929? She'd
had mumps and measles as a child but was terrifically healthy
now—she showed him her biceps, grinning, and the whites of
her eyes.

    And then she turned to him expectantly, pale violet circles
under her eyes, a blameless, indistinct face, as if her features
had been smeared slightly and never clarified, tiny ears, flat

against her head. The whole effect of her was like something that had been started with good intentions and then abandoned out of a sense that what could be created would never be good enough. "What about you?"

"Wait a minute," he said. "Don't go anywhere."

He ran back to the Café de la Paix, took two bottles of beer and a small sack of black walnuts from the kitchen, handed some bills to tall, complacent Trudi, Trudi with an athletic build like a marathoner and a head slightly too small for her magnificent body, who showed people regally to their tables in her shimmering silk hostess dresses — sour-apple green, watermelon. "Going on a date?" she called back to him, and then he ran back to the baby house.

He handed a bottle to Louise, who sat calmly in the dusk, swinging one leg over the other, the light of her cigarette like a stationary insect holding steady before her face, and then he cracked open a walnut and pried out the meat for her.

What about him?

He found he could tell her things — all true — about the farm in Pharaoh, about his uncle's spring (dried up now, but he didn't tell her that), about the bank of blue irises by the stone wall of the barn, about the swarms of swallows crossing the fields at night in fall.

And then — he didn't even have to ask her — she told him about the babies. How many there were. Which ones she nursed: Joseph, Jacob, Bette, Eugene, Nick. She told him that one baby had died. (It was terrible; Alice Vernon was so upset. The parents came. She'd cried, too — they all had — feeling so sorry for them.)

And, he'd never guess — she took a swallow from her beer bottle — one came in, the other day, *in a hatbox.*

How did he like that! She was triumphant, to be the bearer of such news.

So. There it was. St. Louis leaned back against the step behind him and took a deep breath.

Now, whenever he walked past the baby house, the hatbox baby would be there, swaddled tight and laid in its incubator, breathing the special sparkling air, Dr. Hoffman holding a knowing finger to the child's tiny chest, feeling its heartbeat, looking into its eyes with a little light, tapping its skull, communicating the news: *Here you are, your father is dead, I'll look after you now, everything will be all right* . . . or not.

St. Louis realized that he was responsible, in a way, for saving the child's life. First him, and now Hoffman, as if they had agreed to the chain of events, passing the baby from St. Louis's hands to Hoffman's: *You take it from here.*

"I'd like to help those babies," St. Louis said suddenly.

Louise helped herself to another walnut. "That's nice."

He looked down at the stones at his feet. "No, really. I'd like to do something for them."

"Well, unless you got a pair of these"—Louise pointed at her chest, rolled her eyes, giggled.

It was time to go in. She had another feeding at ten. She stood up and stretched. Her dress clung to her big, loose backside in the heat; she picked it free discreetly. She took a little bottle from her purse, sprayed perfume over her neck. "Alice doesn't like us to smoke."

Capuchin the monkey and the organ-grinder came down the dark, empty street behind a street cleaner with his mop and bucket, who was spreading water that smelled of vegetables over the stones. The monkey danced at the end of his leash; the organ-grinder whistled a familiar tune through the curtain of his black mustache. A bitter smell preceded them, burned peanuts, burned oil. The organ-grinder lifted a hand from the handle of his cart, raised his red fez; the monkey shivered and jumped. "Come here, come on," the old man said, reining in the monkey, his voice trailing away as they turned the corner. "Come here, little Capu."

"See you later." Louise stood, flicking her eyes around, reluctant. There were so many things to see, weren't there? Didn't he love Bozo, the roller coaster shaped like a Chinese dragon? Didn't he love the Thrill House of Crime? Didn't he love the darling Cape Cod cottage or the Florida house with its rooftop garden overlooking Lake Michigan? Didn't he love the diamond-cutting exhibit at Lebolt's Jewelers? Didn't he love the fireworks and the diorama of Niagara Falls and the display of beautiful baby cribs at the Lullaby Furniture Company's display, and Aunt Jemima at the Quaker Oats booth?

Of course he did.

"Well, thanks for the beer."

He bowed deeply. "You're doing a good thing, Louise," he told her. "Feeding these babies."

She shrugged. "I get paid."

"But you're helping them. It's important."

She snapped her purse. "I guess that's right. They're sweet. Kind of ugly, in a way, but sweet. I don't mind."

"Good night."

"Good night."

Good night, hatbox baby, he thought, after she had gone inside and he was alone again. And then he went away to sleep.

Dr. Hoffman was waiting for Caro.

He made his last rounds Monday night, finishing at eleven-thirty. The dead boy's baby, he was glad to see, had gained al-

most eleven grams in just these first few days; Alice had bathed
the infant and rubbed it with oil that afternoon. She had made
a note in the baby's chart: "Strong reflexes, good color." It slept
while Dr. Hoffman turned it gently to listen to its heart, pal-
pated its stomach, and looked over the temperature readings
on its chart. It slept with a soundness that felt to Dr. Hoffman
like an adult form of dedication, as if it knew it had to sleep.
He paused over the baby as he put away his stethoscope. *Who's
your mother?* he asked silently in his head. *Who will come
claim you, my friend? You're shaping up to be a record-breaker.
What a shame there is no one here but us to see this.*

And foolish Mrs. Taft, he thought, *would see you taken away
from here, from me.*

Alice was in the back room, measuring vials of breast milk,
when he went in to put away his soiled gown.

"Good night," he said cautiously. He had not told Alice about
his dinner Saturday night with Dr. Ludwig and the Tafts, but
he suspected that she had found out something about it anyway. And she had been enraged by the letter in the newspaper
Sunday morning.

"Does no one call here to check on the facts? Do they not
care about the truth?" She had been indignant, standing before him, the newspaper folded into a tight baton in her hand,
while he drank his coffee at his desk earlier that day and read
over the nurses' charts from the night before. He had been surprised, when he looked up, to see that she was near tears.

"I don't think it's anything to worry about," he'd replied, as
mildly as he could.

Alice had stared at him incredulously. He had decided that
she looked more than upset; she looked almost incandescent
with suppressed rage, as if whatever other sort of ordinary con-
cerns she'd ever had in the world—what to eat, when to sleep,

whether to buy a new hat, or have her shoes resoled or not —
had been burned up in the furnace of her long history of obli-
gation and duty. *All these babies*, he almost heard her say. *All
my babies.*

He'd frowned at her. When had she last had a rest? A proper
vacation?

He'd taken off his glasses. "Alice, we are one of the most
popular . . . exhibits"—he'd had to use the word—"at the fair.
People stream in here. You see them, every day. Nobody thinks
we're doing the babies harm. For goodness sake. There is this
one . . . woman. Her views are, of course, ridiculous. No one
will side with her. Please . . ."

But he could not think exactly what to ask her to do—calm
down? Yes, that, certainly. But more, he'd wanted her to contain herself, to not be so . . . vulnerable. He counted on Alice
to be without extremes, to be full of foresight and common
sense. How old was she? He had to calculate—their fifteen
years together . . . she must be approaching sixty. How long
ago had her brother died, the one she'd lived with? At least
three, maybe four years ago. He had given her a month off after
her brother's death—they'd had no one else but each other—
but she had come back to work after four days. "I'm happier
here," she'd told him. "I don't know what to do with myself at
home. There is nothing to do there."

"Alice." He looked at her back as she stood there now, and
he carefully measured his response. Seeing the cost of her al-
legiance had made him feel grateful and also sad. What would
he have done without her all these years? He knew it was
pointless now to tell her to go to bed, and if he proposed a vacation for her once the fair was over, she would take it as an insult. "Please don't worry," he said instead. "I have been talking
with Dr. Ludwig. I think it will be all right."

But he did not know that. In fact, after that awful dinner—they'd met in a restaurant, over an interminable series of courses ordered in advance by Dr. Ludwig: bouillon and celery and olives, scallops with tartar sauce, roast larded fillet of beef, string beans, candied sweet potatoes, lettuce and chicory salad, ices and cakes, cheese, coffee and demitasse; he'd felt ill from it all—after that awful dinner he had mostly felt the lack of Dr. Ludwig's support. Dr. Ludwig had been mild with Mrs. Taft—a thin, unhappy-looking woman, her head with its short bangs fitted in the back with a hairpiece of shiny curls, her fingers, under an avalanche of diamonds, raw with some skin disorder. Dr. Ludwig had been too mild, Hoffman had thought. Clearly Dr. Ludwig had been dismayed by Mrs. Taft's lack of susceptibility, as he would have called it, to Dr. Hoffman's charms, let alone his own or anyone else's. Her husband, whose bald, domed head shone in the candlelight and whose collar darkened with sweat as the night wore on, had been virtually silent the entire meal. When the talk had finally, after an interminable time spent discussing the weather, sailing on Lake Michigan, Roosevelt and his forgettable vice president, John Garner, Einstein's defection from Germany, the disturbing behavior of the German Nazis, building pyres of books and setting them afire—after all that, finally, Dr. Ludwig had leaned over to refill Mrs. Taft's glass. She had leaned forward, clamping a hand over the rim. Dr. Ludwig carefully returned the bottle to the ice.

"I would trust my own children with my friend Leo Hoffman, Mrs. Taft—Anne, if I may," he began. "I don't know a better doctor, nor one who has contributed more to our understanding of . . ."

But after that, Dr. Hoffman had felt himself drift away from the conversation. He had known it was no good trying to please her or persuade her of anything. Even Dr. Ludwig, smooth, careful, handsome, sincere Dr. Ludwig, would have no effect on her. She was clearly resentful of having been made to come to dinner, and angry with her husband. Dr. Hoffman thought he could picture the unpleasant evening ahead of the poor man after they returned home.

"Well, I certainly won *her* over," he had said to Dr. Ludwig as they waited for their hats after dinner.

"Don't be foolish," Dr. Ludwig had snapped at him.

Dr. Hoffman had taken his hat silently, pushed a dollar tip over the little counter for the hat girl.

"I'm sorry," Dr. Ludwig had said as they left the restaurant and came out into the night air of the street, close and muggy. "I took a risk for you tonight, Leo. They are not people I am inclined to disappoint. They give a great deal of money to my hospital." He sighed. "I can find out who her friends are, where she expects to find support. But do not joke with me about this, please. I have affiliated myself with you because we are old friends, and I do not lie about my esteem for you — you know that. But this is very delicate business."

"I'm sorry." Dr. Hoffman felt abashed.

But though he had tried to make himself think about what lay ahead for his work at the fair that summer, about how he could protect himself, he could not concentrate.

Would she be in his garden when he returned home? Would she knock at his gate?

"Why are you here?" he'd said into her hair that Saturday night after the dinner with Dr. Ludwig and the abominable Tafts. She'd been sitting in his garden when he pushed open the door from his rooms. He had not been able to stop himself from putting his arms around her almost at once—the relief of it, that she was there.

"I don't know," she had said, but he had not minded the obvious honesty of her answer to his question.

They had not spoken much. He had, at last, let her go, unknotted his tie, unbuttoned the cuffs of his shirtsleeves, poured them each a glass of wine. Then they sat across from each other, their knees interlaced, and he held her hands, or ran his palms up her arms and over her shoulders, touched her face, her hair, kissed her. The strangeness of her presence there with him, the unlikeliness of it, only enhanced his feeling of ease and license—it wasn't entirely real, that he should be allowed to touch this woman, this woman he barely knew, this woman to whom he'd been yoked, as he'd thought of it before, in such an unfortunate way. He had thought her a discredit, thought her proximity an insult. It made him want to laugh, how such a trick, such a good joke, had been played on him. He did laugh. He held her face in his hands and kissed her and laughed. She had seemed mild, almost surprised, he thought later, lying alone in his sheets. He thought he understood that, too. The surprise of it.

He had worried she would never return, but she had come back Sunday night, too. He'd poured her more wine, plied her with questions. Where had she been born? Who were her parents? He did not ask about her dancing, but he asked where she had traveled, what cities she had liked best. What she did when she was not at work.

And finally, he took her to bed.

Afterward, he lay in the dark with his arms around her, relishing the smell and feel of her beside him.

"And you are all alone here?" he asked at last.

"My cousin is with me," she said, rolling over to face him. "We were raised together."

"Your cousin?"

She shrugged inside his embrace, as if she could not explain the relationship any further. "He's like a brother."

"What does he do?"

"Well"—Caro had laughed—"he looks after us. He looks after the money. We keep each other company."

"And his name?" Hoffman was polite.

Caro laughed again. "St. Louis," she said.

Hoffman raised his eyebrows.

"For the city, not the saint," Caro said. "He was born there." She seemed to be remembering. "He was a premature baby, like . . . yours. And then his mother—my aunt—left him with us." She paused. "He *is* a saint, in a way, though. He's short, like a dwarf." She put out her hand, palm down, several feet from the floor beside Hoffman's bed, as if this St. Louis might appear there beside them, the top of his head grazing her fingers.

"I see."

"I see," he'd said, but it was a mechanical answer. *I see your face,* he'd thought, *your lips and your hair and your body.* He'd put his hands on her back and pulled her near him so that her face, when it came close to his, presented itself with a complete and willing acquiescence. The slight pillow of her cheek was like nothing so much as what it was, a beautiful woman's profile, powdered, scented, soft, desirable, a perfect curve.

On Monday night, Alice stood in the nursery's back room with her back to him, a slight trickle of cold water leaking with a dismal sound into the sink. She held up her hand, silently asking him to wait a minute. Alice could not speak when measuring things; he knew that about her. He did not really want to discuss Mrs. Taft's insulting letter again—that foolish woman's letter. And it was impossible to comfort Alice. But he didn't feel he could leave. She clearly wanted to talk. He was impatient—would Caro be in his rooms again? But he waited until Alice had finished.

Alice turned around at last, wiped her hands. "I want to show you something," she said.

Dr. Hoffman followed her back out into the nursery. Alice had dimmed the lights. The four nurses on duty were busy cleaning thermometers and bottles or tending to the babies. Alice led him over to the incubator that housed the baby C. K. From a shelf under the baby's incubator, she withdrew a small box. "Look," she said, and opened the top.

Inside, on a bed of cotton, was a gold coin. Dr. Hoffman leaned over. He did not recognize the denomination or the origin of the coin. It looked old. He picked it up and examined it.

"I found it in his incubator," Alice said. "The grandmother put it in there."

Dr. Hoffman frowned, rubbing at the surface of the coin with his thumb. "What is it?"

"I think it's for good luck. You know, like a medal."

Dr. Hoffman handed it back to her.

"It was *inside* his gown." Alice closed the box over it and leaned down to put it away again.

Dr. Hoffman looked in at C. K. "What do they stand for?" he asked suddenly. "The initials."

Alice turned to him. "They stand for Charles, I think, some version of Charles. And then something else—I can't pronounce it. I can't understand the grandmother very well, and the mother is still too ill to visit." She waited a moment. "What do you want me to do?" she asked finally.

Dr. Hoffman turned to her. He raised his eyebrows.

"About the *grandmother*." Alice's tone was impatient.

"About the grandmother?" He thought for a minute. "Well, I assume you have cleaned everything. The bedding, the gown—"

"Yes, of course." Alice glared at him.

Hoffman opened the doors to the incubator. He reached in and put a hand on C. K. The baby, one of the larger infants, at three and a half pounds, stirred. One of its arms, freed from its wrapper, jerked upward in a frantic swimming motion. "Excuse me," Hoffman said to the baby. "I have woken you up now, and Alice had just settled you for the night." He tucked the baby's arm back inside the gown, turned the infant on its side. He patted the child's back. The baby's lower extremities were disturbingly stiff, but it did not appear to be a worsening condition. Spastic diplegia, Dr. Hoffman thought. If he lived, he'd be lucky to walk.

"Dr. Hoffman."

He turned around to face Alice again.

"What do you want to say to the grandmother?"

"I don't want to say anything to her," he said. "Of course she can't bring such things in here. You will tell her so and show her that you keep the medal—or the coin, whatever it is—under the incubator." He raised his eyebrows again.

Alice looked away from him, unsatisfied.

"What's the matter?" he said. "The damage is done already. If there is to be microbic infection transmitted to the baby from his grandmother's . . . good luck charm, there is nothing we can do except treat it when it appears."

"Yes, I know. I know."

She looked away from him and stared in at C. K. "I don't like it," she said suddenly.

Dr. Hoffman waited.

"I can't account for it, but I'm worried."

"You are tired," he began. "Go get some rest."

She shook her head.

Dr. Hoffman put his hand on her shoulder. "It's César," he said. "You hate to lose them."

But Alice turned to him then. "I wish I felt better," she said. "I know it doesn't make sense, and I wouldn't say it to anybody but you. But I just have a bad feeling."

Dr. Hoffman kept his hand on her shoulder for a minute and frowned at her. "We are all tired," he said.

Alice sighed. "Yes. Yes, we are all tired."

Dr. Hoffman turned her around and pushed her gently toward the door, helping her out of her gown as they went. "You will feel better in the morning," he said. "I'm sure of it."

But Alice didn't answer him directly. She dropped her gown in the laundry bin and waited for him at the door to the nursery.

Dr. Hoffman put both hands on her shoulders when they were in the hall. "There is no better nurse," he said.

She gave a small smile. "Well . . ."

"Good night," he called as she walked away.

But Alice only raised her hand behind her.

Caro was not in his rooms when he opened the door.

He checked his pocket watch. It would still be early for her perhaps. She would not be ready until after midnight. He was just as glad to have a minute to think. It was not like Alice to be irrational. She rarely said such things to him. But her instincts as a nurse were excellent, as good as his own. He wished she had not chosen tonight to voice such vague worries. He did not want to think about anything else going wrong.

He set his watch beside the bed, changed his shirt, washed his face, and shaved, and then, with still a half hour to go before Caro might reasonably be expected to arrive, he made himself sit in the garden and read a long letter from a physician in Paris who wanted Hoffman to review, before its publication, a lecture on the adaptations made by Asiatic Eskimos for prolonging the lives of infants born too soon. The Eskimos, Hoffman read, put their premature babies into the whole skins of seabirds that had been gutted and then turned inside out, with the feathers inside. The infants were bound within this soft, supple skin and then suspended over a low flame and fed doses of oil (*What sort?* Hoffman wondered, making a note in the margin) mixed with breast milk. Hoffman's colleague in Paris was speculating on the efficacy of oil administered to infants too weak to suckle as an antidote to apnea attacks while feeding. Hoffman bent over the table and pulled his candle closer.

"What are you reading?"

He looked up with a start. She was standing beside him, in the same clothes she'd worn the night he'd caught her swimming in Lake Michigan, a man's pair of khaki trousers, a man's white shirt. She was smiling as if she had planned to startle him. Her hair was pinned close at her neck but then fell down her back. *Blackberry,* he thought. *China black.*

He jumped up and took her hands. "I am so glad to see you."

She leaned into him when he kissed her. When he let her go, she ran a hand through her hair, pulled out a chair, and sat down. "What are you reading? May I have a glass of wine?"

"Of course." He left the terrace and went inside. Dr. Ludwig's cook, who came by every night with a cold supper for him, had left a plate of ham and biscuits, a bowl of nectarines, and a plate of éclairs under a net in the tiny pantry; the surface of the pastry was stiff with a sugar glaze, as if the éclairs had been painted to the plate. He had a sudden instinct to look at a clock, though there was none, only his watch by the bed. How long had he been reading? What time was it? He put the éclairs aside, covering them with a napkin, and brought the bowl instead, a bottle of champagne under his arm, and in his other hand a bunch of red roses, purchased early that morning for her and held in the sink filled halfway with water. The petals had already begun to drop, dismaying him.

She took the bowl of fruit from him to set it on the table and smiled when he handed her the roses. She held the bouquet to her face. "St. Louis gets them from one of the gardeners at the Horticulture Building. Did you know that someone has bred a nearly black rose? He brought me some the other day. I thought they were awful."

"It doesn't seem a very good color for a flower."

"No. But I gather they've been trying for some time. It was apparently quite a triumph."

Hoffman smiled at her. He uncorked the champagne and poured them each a glass. He would be tired in the morning, he thought briefly. And champagne sometimes gave him a headache.

"What were you reading?" she asked him again.

He looked down at the closely covered pages on the table. "An article. From a colleague."

She took a sip of her champagne. "What's it about?"

He glanced at her. "Are you really interested? It's rather obscure."

"I am."

He told her briefly about the Eskimos, but he did not attempt to make it interesting. These two things, Caro and the babies—they did not really belong together. He leaned forward and touched his champagne glass to hers. "Can I tell you," he said, interrupting himself, "how"—he had to laugh; he shook his head—"how you make me . . . speechless?" He blushed. It sounded rehearsed, but he had meant it.

He could not see his own face then, of course, only hers, but he understood—with a kind of thrill that was like standing up at the top of a mountain and seeing for the first time a view so much talked about—the caliber of her response to him, the dreadful, shining truth of it. No matter what happened—and he was aware of the acres of deceit that could lie ahead of them—no matter what happened—he knew even that they might one day be forgotten to each other, though the thought sent a current of grief through him that he imagined aged him a year in just a split second—*still, no matter what happened,* nothing would change this one moment, when he knew she loved him.

She would not say so, though. He marveled that he knew this, too, Leo Hoffman, a man with so little experience. And then, just as he could sometimes see the course of a baby's life ahead of it, with an apprehension both precise and yet global, the almost vertiginous perspective he was sometimes capable of, he thought he knew what would happen next, and he felt himself stiffen.

"Would you take me to see your babies?"

He set his glass down and leaned over without looking at her to put his arms around her. "What do you want to see the babies for?" he asked, though he could guess; it had all been there in that look she'd worn a moment ago.

She shrugged within his arms.

What could he say to her? That he could not come walking

into his nursery in the middle of the night with her. He could not . . . show her around. What would his nurses think? Dr. Ludwig's resident—what was his name? Dr. Sandor? What would he think?

"I can't," he said finally. He kissed her hair, sorry.

"Hundreds of people see them, every day. Only just a few less than come to see me." She pulled away from him, but she was smiling.

Embarrassed, he reached behind him for the bottle to refill their glasses.

She watched him. "You will not take me there in the middle of the night because it's irregular. I understand. But tomorrow? During the day?"

"Why do you want to see them so much?"

She paused. "I don't know. I'm interested."

He thought for a moment. "And you are interested, too, in whether *I* will take you. Because you could go for twenty-five cents yourself, of course." He was sorry as soon as he'd said it—it sounded brutal and unkind. What made him sound so haughty?

She looked up at him, as if surprised that he would say this out loud, though she did not seem injured by it.

He reached out again and took her fingers. "Did you see the letter in the newspaper?" He looked down at her hand, massaging the joints of her fingers.

She was quiet for a moment. "St. Louis read it to me."

He nodded.

"Is it the first time you've had such objections raised against you?" she asked.

"Against me, personally—yes. Others who deserved to be shut down have been publicly exposed, though not here."

"Not in the United States?"

"No. There is no one else in the United States who does what I do."

He didn't like the sound of how that had come out, either; it sounded pompous, and he had meant it only as a statement of fact. There was silence between them for a few moments, and then she stood up and stretched. He looked up at her but did not move to pull her back toward him. He had not wanted to think about any of this. He had wanted to sleep with her again. It had been so wonderful, and tonight especially, with Alice's grim warning in his head, he wanted her.

She stood looking down at him. "Are you worried about it?"

"I'm not sure," he said. "I don't know what to make of it exactly."

She came toward him then. She tipped his face up toward her and kissed him deeply on the mouth. "It wasn't a nice letter," she said. "I'm sorry."

He put his hands up to make her stay, but she bent again and kissed him quickly. "Someday," she said, "maybe you will show me your babies."

And then she opened his gate and disappeared into the street.

It would have been easy to overreact and tell himself she would never be back, but he thought that wasn't true and his saying so would be mostly a result of his own sexual disappointment at that moment. Because he thought she *would* be back. He had not been wrong about that look on her face, he thought. Gathering up their glasses and the bowl of fruit, he paused. *Amazing,* he thought, *that I feel so sure of that.*

But as he stepped inside, into the pitch dark of his bedroom —the smell of cedar, the sour scent of his own dirty shirts, the sweet scent of lilies in a vase, flowers with sticky brown pollen that soiled his hands, the smell of *her,* still, from yesterday and the day before—he remembered something. *"That such unfortunate babes are to be exhibited alongside fat women, catchpenny monstrosities, fire walkers, and fan dancers"*—oh God —*"should and does offend our deepest sense of integrity and charity."*

Now he remembered that, the insult to her. But he had not remembered it in time.

He sat down on the bed, putting the bowl at his feet. He had not imagined this sort of pain, he thought at first—the knowledge that he had wounded her. And then it came to him, practically as he had this thought, that in fact he *did* recognize it—hadn't his parents hurt each other in precisely this way? His mother had been so intelligent, so passive, with her large eyes, her smooth hair, her still hands, her genius for mathematics that would, in the end, earn her the love of her pupils but not the admiration of her colleagues. His father had been the greater of the two of them, the more powerful, the more confident. He had walked about all the time with the knowledge of his own superiority secure in his breast pocket; *that* was what had hurt her, that he had needed to always protect himself from her in that way. He could easily have paved her way into prestigious academic circles, Dr. Hoffman thought now. Women needed sponsors from men in the professional world. But he had never opened that door to her. He had needed to keep her shut out, perhaps because, at an important level, he was not brave enough to include her.

And now he too would divide Caro from himself—from his babies—because he felt he *had* to.

His chest ached. He would have given, at that moment, almost anything to have Caro beside him. Now he remembered his father's face, looking out at his mother as she walked in the garden or sat with a book by herself. He had loved her, Dr.

Hoffman thought, remembering his father's grave, sad face. His father had loved her.

But maybe not enough.

It was worse than one's own injury, he thought, for which one could at least hope for convalescence and recovery, even in the midst of the worst of the agony.

It was hurting her that would kill him, he realized now with wonderment.

And now he already had.

Chicago

August 1933

◼

TEN

On Monday, August 28, a set of triplet boys was born to Mrs. Winnie and Mr. Paul Fusco, residents of Chicago, Mr. Fusco being employed in a butcher's shop on the North Side as a meat carver, and his wife as a part-time dressmaker by the department stores Marshall Field's and Goldblatt's and Wieboldt's, where she rotated from one thickly carpeted dressing room to the next, on her knees performing alterations to men's cuffs and waistbands, their shirtsleeves and inseams. Mr. Fusco was mustached and tended to be fat, though neither money nor food was plentiful: Jobless men lined the curbs, the bailiff's office evicted thousands of families each year that were unable to pay the rent, banks closed their doors by the dozens. Squatters tied up their houseboats to the shores of the north branch of the Chicago River, and in the reeking villages of the unemployed on Canal Street, built of flattened tin cans and tar paper and scrap lumber, the citizens erected flagpoles at the mud-filled intersections of what passed for main thoroughfares through the shacks. Poverty had begun to take on an air of desolate permanence.

But Mr. Fusco seemed to increase helplessly in size even when his portions were diminished. His hair had retreated early in his thirties, leaving a tonsure surrounded by red curls like sea foam, which he pressed hopelessly to his head in times of high anxiety. During the birth of his sons—an event that took both him and his wife by surprise, for she was not due to deliver for another seven weeks—he stood by the bed with his hands glued to his head, a posture that gave him the air of an astonished bystander who had simply stumbled upon a woman giving birth, first to one baby and then another and then, at last, to a third.

The tiny babies came fast, sluicing out of Mrs. Fusco following a ferocious cramping just before dawn. This was her first pregnancy, and she mistook the pains at first for indigestion. Though she had seen a doctor twice since determining that she was pregnant, no one had suggested she might be carrying twins, let alone triplets. Between the second and third delivery, Winnie rolled over, weeping, to be held by Mr. Fusco, who knelt by the bed now, his sleeves rolled up, helping the babies out from between his wife's legs, though his hands always seemed to be in the way somehow. The babies were an unusual color, the blue-gray of a stormy sky, and made no sound. They lay on the sheets, wrapped in towels, twitching. Winnie Fusco's fingers, when Mr. Fusco held her hands, were dry and stiff as cardboard, perforated with tiny white blisters and scars from a lifetime's encounter with the needle. The skin around her lips and thin nose was white as chalk. "Not the doctor, the priest," she whispered. "Get the priest."

The baby boys, baptized at Winnie's bedside by the sweating priest down the street at St. Paul's, who had been interrupted at his breakfast of coffee and leftover yellow cake by a boy of ten sent at a run down Pulaski Road to fetch him, were named Lawrence, Emerson, and Marshall. Immediately after the priest's departure—the trembling father's apologetic white hands, silky as flour, slipping away at last from the babies' wet, blue-black foreheads—the infants were taken to the fairgrounds of the Century of Progress by Mr. Fusco and his friend and employer, Mr. Bernini, who was, fortunately, the owner of a car and had been to see the incubator exhibit at the Century of Progress the week before.

Mr. Fusco sat in the backseat of the car, and Mrs. Bernini, smoking a cigarette in her distress and dropping ash on Mr. Fusco's shirtfront, ran up and down the stairs fetching babies and handing them in to Mr. Fusco. As the car pulled away in a puff of gray exhaust, she felt the palms of her hands burning, as though God had slapped her there for feeling afraid. After the car disappeared, she stood outside on the street for a moment, feeling behind her the quiet apartment building with its patterned carpet leading up the stairs and through the kitchenette and into the bedroom. Mrs. Bernini, who had no children herself, had never seen anything so terrifying as those tiny babies.

She and Mr. Bernini had only come by to pick up Mr. Fusco for work. Now she felt she'd had a terrifying brush with the . . . beginning of things. The impossible to imagine.

Why had none of them thought to get a doctor? Or call for an ambulance? It was so odd, she thought—two babies already on the bed when they arrived, and the third coming, and the priest arriving and her husband, Sal, saying that about the baby doctor at the fair . . . Well, it was done now.

Mrs. Bernini lit another cigarette and plucked at the bosom of her dress, lifting the damp cloth away from the stickiness of her skin. It felt to her like God had lit a furnace in the sky.

The heat had indeed deepened over the summer, the bright, electric blaze of June followed by the thick temperatures of July, when moss inched over trees in Washington Park and strange rings of white mushrooms appeared in the grass. The jobless men sitting in the Old Peristyle in Grant Park and reading the papers for want ads gave off a smoky vapor, as if the heat were burning them up and turning them to dust. Lake Michigan glittered, and the fairgrounds, as the sun reached its zenith, hovered behind rippling waves of heat. In August, thunderstorms rolling west to east across the country shook the trees and broke branches and whipped up funnels of water in the lake. But the storms left behind only a citywide sense of failure and stupefaction. Those who were desperate, those sliding further into poverty, and those few lucky enough to be modestly secure—all seemed to suffer the oppression of the weather. By dawn, whatever poor amount of rain had fallen during the night had passed, and the streets would be searing again by ten. People's joints ached from the turbulence of the barometer. Cats wailed on ridgepoles. Locusts sawed in the fields, goods tumbled from the shelves in the groceries, and pearls in jewelers' velvet cases acquired a milky film that could not be rubbed away with a cloth. Mae West's film *She Done Him Wrong* slipped from the reels of projectors in the popcorn palaces of the movie houses, unwinding with the sound of things gone haywire.

It was eleven in the morning when Mr. Bernini nosed the car over the Michigan Avenue bridge. The Lindbergh beacon in the Palmolive Building glowed red-hot in the haze. Twenty feet under Mr. Bernini's tires, on the lower level of the bridge, homeless men slept through the morning in piles of manure dust, covered with a film fine as fallen ash.

When Mr. Bernini arrived at last at the gates to the fair, he had to raise his voice in anger before he succeeded in finally seeing the gates opened to admit the car, the ticket taker retreating fast, as if he had smelled something bad, after venturing to stick his head in the rear window to be certain that there were, as Mr. Bernini had insisted, three tiny, desperate babies back there.

Mr. Bernini drove carefully through the crowds, which parted sluggishly ahead of his fender; clots of people turned to stare resentfully through the automobile's windows at Mr. Fusco's burning, mortified face—who did he think *he* was? Mr. Fusco held the babies bunched in his arms. His spine gave out a dull, steady ache, his bowels sloshing dangerously, liquid and hot.

But when the car reached the Streets of Paris, Mr. Bernini could go no further. The crowd was so thick that he did not think even a child could slip through it. People were stacked up in the street, craning over one another's heads, pressing one another's shoulders in order to get a better view. He turned around and peered back at Mr. Fusco, who searched the heads and shoulders out the window and then turned back to his friend with an expression of dismay.

Mr. Bernini assessed the situation. "I'll see what . . ." He got out of the car with difficulty; there were so many people in the street he couldn't open the door all the way. Already three young men had climbed to the DeSoto's hot, shiny roof.

"Get down from there!" He waved his arms to shoo them away, but no one moved.

Inside the car, Mr. Fusco bent over his babies. Mr. Bernini's shirt flattened stickily once against the window, the hair embroidering the white flesh of his back visible through the soaked cloth of his shirt. He peeled away and then was pressed back.

"Please," Mr. Fusco heard Mr. Bernini say, "I'm trying to get to the doctor. I have a man with three little babies here, we need to get to the incubator doctor, I have—"

But then Mr. Fusco could hear no more, as Mr. Bernini's voice was drowned out by a wave of laughter in the crowd outside. He heard a sudden drum roll, a clash of cymbals, the sound of a woman's affronted yelp; he heard screams, and then the crowd roared again.

"What is it?" Mr. Bernini was bewildered; he cast about wildly. People were screaming with laughter; some were applauding. "What's going on?"

"Here." A man who was crouched on top of Mr. Bernini's car leaned down and offered Mr. Bernini a hand, and as Mr. Bernini felt himself being pulled up, as easily and effortlessly as if he weighed nothing more than a leaf, onto the smooth black roof of his car, one of the babies—it was Marshall, the smallest—stiffened suddenly in Mr. Fusco's arms inside the car, reared up on the base of his spine like a sea horse, and shook violently. The baby's mouth opened, its tiny nostrils flared, and its eyes, which had been squeezed shut, rolled open once to reveal what looked, to the horrified Mr. Fusco, like an empty nothingness, a ghastly, blank white marble, the moon pinched from the sky and set to rolling in his son's eye socket. And then the child was utterly still.

"Sal." Mr. Fusco's voice was something squeezed out of a clenched fist. "Help."

But Salvator Bernini was staring in amazement down the street from his position on the roof of the car.

In front of a big pink building, which he recognized as the incubator exhibit, a circle of four massive gray elephants, their absurd tails like little willow switches held in the loose grasp of one another's wrinkled trunks, paraded slowly. By the elephants' heads strode four dark-skinned men in white turbans and black tailcoats and billowing pantaloons in burning shades of cadmium yellow and crimson and ultramarine, their cuffs trimmed with gold ribbon and tiny silver bells. A band of midget musicians dressed in Bavarian lederhosen and sky blue blouses, playing cymbals and drums and pennywhistles, darted in and out between the elephants' mighty, slow-moving legs. And protesting on the elephants backs, embraced by four more graceful men in turbans, their white teeth showing, were four matronly women in careful suit dresses and tiny hats and short veils. Two of them were white as sheets; one screamed unintelligibly and tried to fight off her captor; and one beat weakly at her elephant's massive and distant shoulder with a cardboard placard that had been mounted on a small wooden post the size and heft of a child's school ruler.

Inside the car, Mr. Fusco's hand moved tentatively down inside the blanket that held Emerson, now one of his two remaining sons. Mr. Fusco's big hand—the skin smooth as stone from having kneaded so much animal fat and pliable strings of muscle and sinew, the fingers strong and probing, able to snap a joint—gently touched the baby's chest. Mr. Fusco's eyes were closed, his lips moving in prayer. With one finger he traced the cords of the little neck, thin as a belt loop, it seemed, down to the baby's chest, which rose and fell rapidly.

Fifty-five breaths per minute, sixty breaths per minute, Dr. Hoffman would have said, counting by instinct, if he'd been there holding the child, if they'd ever been able to reach the hospital. The shallow agonal breaths of a baby in respiratory distress.

The baby took two, three, four deep, gasping sighs, the tiny chest surging away like a darting minnow's back under Mr. Fusco's quivering fingertip and then rising one last time. And then nothing.

There was nothing Dr. Hoffman could have done anyway.

The crowd pressed up against the car, blocking the light.

Mr. Fusco saw the checkered pattern of a woman's dress loom up by his ear, her bulging hip and bosom. He saw the white shirts of many men. A pair of scuffed brown heels drummed against the car window nearest his head; the car sank once on its tires, then bounced as someone slipped from the roof.

It was Mr. Bernini, whose face appeared anxiously over the headrest.

"They're dying." Mr. Fusco put his palms instinctively over the faces of his two dead children, as if to grant them privacy. "Two of them are dead already, Sal."

Mr. Bernini knelt on the seat, looked down at the babies in Mr. Fusco's arms. "I'm sorry," he whispered, and then together they watched the third and last baby, named Lawrence for Mrs. Fusco's father. And as they watched, Lawrence repeated his brother Emerson's last moments, as if he had only been waiting courteously for him to finish before taking his place in the queue—the same rapid breathing, the same deep, final gasps, and then nothing.

"Oh," said Mr Fusco, and he began to weep openly. "Oh, Sal. What am I going to tell Winnie? What do I tell Winnie?"

Mr. Bernini turned around slowly and sat staring out the windshield, his hands cupped over the steering wheel. The crowd had now begun to thin around them, breaking apart. Far ahead he could see the retreating haunches of the last elephant moving away, a pile of rock.

"I couldn't get through," he said to Mr. Fusco, who sat behind him, his lap full of the lifeless babies, his arms trying to contain them. "It was some kind of demonstration. Some women protesting the incubator exhibit. And then"—he shook his head—"and then the guy said these elephants came along and they just *scooped*"—and his voice rose incredulously— "they *scooped* up the women and—." He stopped and then hit

the steering wheel twice with his hands. "*Protesting* the doctor!" he said. "Protesting a *doctor*. Goddamn. Goddamn."

Dr. Hoffman had not expected Alice to be pleased by
what had happened that morning—that preposterous scene
with the elephants. But she had been. He had refused to go
outside during the commotion, either to confront the protesters
themselves or to see them borne away by the elephants. A
month ago he might have had a taste for it, for a kind of re-
venge. But not anymore. Not now.

He'd been waiting for Mrs. Taft to appear picketing one day,
though; her letters, which had been increasing in their vehe-
mence, had promised as much, and he was not surprised when
the man delivering canisters of oxygen earlier that morning had
reported the ladies' presence outside. Dr. Hoffman had felt only
a tired acknowledgment at the news. Did they think he had
been worrying about them? He did not care anything for them.

But Alice had gone out immediately when one of the wet
nurses—forgetting herself entirely—had come squealing into
the nursery with the news that a parade of elephants was outside and had come and picked up the ladies with the signs!

When Alice and Nan Silverman and three of the other nurses
had come back inside a half hour later, Dr. Hoffman had been
listening to little Helen's lungs. The faint, wet crackles he had
imagined he'd heard the night before, the sure warning sign of
pneumonia, were not present this morning. Now the baby's
breath came sweetly to him, the smooth, reassuring sound of
wind in a willow tree. But last night, when he had picked her
up and made a V of his fingers to press the stethoscope to her
chest, the sound of her breathing had terrified him—here it
was again. Here was the thicket he'd been lost in once as a boy,
a dark forest in Germany where his parents had stopped one

holiday for tea and he had gone outside the inn to play. Here were the wet leaves underfoot, here was the strange, enormous bird, startled from the branches overhead, flapping away darkly through the trees into the sky's filthy light. Helen had been so strong. What had happened?

He'd had to wrench the stethoscope out of his ears and back away for a moment to collect himself.

He had lost ten babies now this summer —beginning with poor César Fluvio. Standing there now, weak with relief at Helen's improvement this morning, he realized how great was his fatigue. Complacency would be his lifetime enemy, a failure of character, a vice, like gambling or a tendency to drink. He could never relax. And Alice, Alice with her dire warnings and her bad feelings of earlier this summer—she had been right. He should have listened to her. Though what good would it have done to listen? What could he have done?

The infection that had begun with César Fluvio had spread first to his twin brother. And then eight other babies had sickened and died; three had been simply too small to begin with. Dr. Hoffman wondered now at his once having been so absurdly confident they would survive. The other five had died from an infection whose symptoms resembled those of César's: the sudden high fever, the convulsions. It was impossible to say if it was the same thing or something else altogether.

Despite having quarantined many infants in an effort to prevent the spread of the infection—a move that had meant hiring extra nurses and working to the point of exhaustion those he had brought with him initially—and despite redoubled measures of cleanliness on his part, he had still lost ten babies in eight weeks. Three among them had been infants that Dr. Ludwig had urged him to take, babies born to

Chicagoans. Dr. Hoffman had felt angry at Dr. Ludwig for what he saw as his friend's role in the nursery's failure, though he knew it was foolish to cast blame. Such deaths had occurred before, several infants in a cluster. But never at a fair.

The deaths made a mockery of his ambition of earlier in the summer. The perfect summer, not a single death—had he actually believed he could manage that? When he thought of it now, he felt humiliated.

But for the last two weeks, there had been no new signs of danger. He had begun to take his dinner in his own rooms again instead of in the nursery—with Caro, if she could join him. They sat together, holding hands, and afterward they made a kind of violent love that frightened them both. *I feel like I'm losing you,* he had wanted to say. But he had not spoken. She had given him no sign of diminishing affection, and what he felt—this aching sense of dread—made no sense. What was the point of saying anything about it?

The remaining babies had grown, ounce by steady ounce. He had increased the monitoring and observation to a level even Alice complained had been unnecessary—checking the babies' temperatures, checking their pulses, listening to their hearts, their bowels, their lungs, almost every hour. He himself circled the ward obsessively, hardly leaving the nursery at all during the day and often not at night, either. Moving from incubator to incubator, lifting the babies in his hands one after another and closing his eyes, he could feel the sounds of the lungs and heart in his fingertips—*Here's rain on a roof, here's a mouse caught in a drum*— feel the character and rate of the pulse, feel the skin for the faintest sheen of perspiration or the advancing chill of cyanosis in cold fingers and toes. He had stood with the babies in his arms, his cheek to their mouths to smell their breath and listen to their breathing and their bowels, and had tried to summon up in himself powers that might take him beyond what ordinarily could be heard and seen and felt and on into another realm, a different place, where he sensed prayer was his tool and so applied himself there: *Give me a sign*, he had prayed, the babies' hearts beating under his fingers, their tiny fingers gripped around his own. *At least, give me warning.*

Now, little Helen in his arms, her chest suddenly clear, he was able to greet Alice's return to the nursery with pleasure born of his relief.

He laid Helen back in her incubator, closed the door, and walked over to Alice. "Was it a spectacle?" He put his glasses in his pocket and folded his arms over Helen's chart against his chest.

"I call it a miracle." Alice lifted Robert, the baby with the cleft palate, onto her lap, unfolded his wrapper with expert hands, and began gently massaging his tiny chest with fingers she had first dipped in a cup of sweet almond oil warmed over a burner. She smiled down at the baby, who thrashed ineffectually on her lap. "Go on," she said, encouraging him. "Fight me off. Go on!"

"I think it depends on whose perspective you see it from." Dr. Hoffman looked down at Alice, watching her hands moving expertly over the baby's abdomen.

She turned Robert over like a pancake and began tapping his back. "We've taken good care of *you*, my friend," she said to the baby. "When you grow up, you can go and show yourself to that foolish Mrs. Taft and give her a pop on the nose."

Dr. Hoffman leaned over and put his hand on the baby's head briefly. Under his fingers he felt the split halves of the skull, its rough seam, the baby's throbbing fontanel. He sat down beside Alice, Helen's chart on his lap. Unfolding his glasses and putting them on again, he looked down at his handwriting from the night before. "Who do you suppose managed it?"

Alice bent over Robert. "Lift that head, young man. Go on. I know you can do it."

Dr. Hoffman waited. Alice did not seem to be paying attention to him. "I mean, the elephants didn't just spontaneously come to our rescue," he said finally. "I suppose I am much obliged to them, but it hardly seems an accident."

Alice lifted the baby's arms, gave them a gentle tug. "You know how the fair people are. They like to stick together."

Dr. Hoffman looked up from Helen's chart, but Alice was not looking at him. She made puckering noises with her mouth in the direction of Robert's ear. "La la la, my love. La la la."

"Since when did we become *fair people?*" he said.

"All I know, and all I care about, is that those women— those stupid women—stay away from this hospital." Alice stroked Robert's head. "I don't care if men from the moon come and take them away in flying saucers. I hope they're too embarrassed to come back here with their stupid signs."

Dr. Hoffman regarded Alice for a minute. There was something she wasn't telling him; he could tell by the way she wouldn't look at him directly. Could *she* have arranged such an elaborate interference? He thought not. Maybe it was as she suggested—maybe the women seemed an affront to the entire fair community. He was surprised to consider that he might have friends among his neighbors. He hardly spoke to any of them—except Caro, of course. He made a few last notes in his chart and then sat back. "Shame about his face," he said, reaching a finger toward Robert, stroking the baby's cheek to see him turn his head, the rooting reflex.

Dr. Hoffman had invented a device that allowed Robert to suckle more efficiently—a strip of dental-rubber dam about

two inches wide was placed over the baby's nose and upper lip
and tied tightly to block off the nostrils. In between sucking
contractions the upper edge over the nose was lifted so Robert
could breathe. He was able to get much more milk this way;
the split lip would have made it hard for him to be sufficiently
nourished otherwise. Dr. Hoffman was pleased that the device
had worked so well. Later he could be attended to surgically,
but he was too small now.

"He'll be gorgeous when all's said and done. And he's such a
love . . . aren't you?" Alice's tone was fierce. She flipped the
baby again, wrapped him up, gathering his limbs together
neatly. "You and our wee hatbox baby," she said to the infant.
"You're going to be our record-breakers, aren't you?"

At the mention of the hatbox baby, Dr. Hoffman stood up
and folded Helen's chart closed. He checked his watch. He had
promised to meet Dr. Ludwig for lunch. He had hardly seen
him over the past few weeks. The proliferation of letters in the
newspaper deriding the incubator exhibit had so receded in
his mind, owing to the urgency of his duties in the nursery,
that he had been avoiding Dr. Ludwig. But Dr. Ludwig had
continued to worry him about it, pressing him to attend dinners with the fair board, urging him to grant interviews with a
woman magazine writer Dr. Ludwig had managed to interest in
Dr. Hoffman's story. Dr. Ludwig had annoyed him especially
by coming to the nursery one day in the worst of the crisis with
a photographer and insisting on several photographs of Dr.
Hoffman and Nan Silverman—an attractive woman—he had
specifically *not* asked for Alice—holding the babies.

Nan, under the spell of Dr. Ludwig's charm and insistence,
had hurriedly run a brush through her hair, changed her uniform, and joined Dr. Hoffman—Dr. Ludwig had arranged him
in a rocking chair—with a baby in her arms.

"And who have we here?" Dr. Ludwig had said, taking the baby and settling him cozily in Dr. Hoffman's wooden embrace. "Relax, Dr. Hoffman. You look like a man condemned to death. It's only a photograph."

Nan had spoken up. "We call him the—"

But Dr. Hoffman had interrupted her. For some reason, he had not wanted Dr. Ludwig to know about the hatbox baby's unusual history. The baby's mother had never appeared, and though Dr. Hoffman had not been entirely surprised by this, he had come to realize that the infant's likely status as an orphan weighed upon him with a special anxiety. Yet the child seemed to require almost nothing of his protectors. Despite having been so dehydrated that first day, he'd hated the gavage feedings from the start, reacting with such profound distress that Dr. Hoffman had been worried he would aspirate fluid into his lungs. Instead, he seemed to manage nursing at the breast well enough, growing steadily more competent as the weeks passed. And though he wore out quickly, his pulse rising to dizzying levels—Dr. Hoffman ordered additional feedings instead, shorter in duration—he seemed more comfortable at the breast than feeding any other way. When the other babies had become ill, Dr. Hoffman had moved the hatbox baby into quarantine as well, though he could not explain himself to Alice, who had asked why the baby should require a separate nurse when he wasn't ill, especially when so many others were.

But sometimes Dr. Hoffman would go and sit by the child and simply watch him sleep. The chair by the baby's incubator became, in fact, where Dr. Hoffman took what little rest he could find during the day. In the aura of the baby's steady and silent growth, its lack of struggle or distress, he experienced a sensation of calm himself. From time to time the troubling image of the young man who had been murdered on the street came into his head while he watched the baby; he thought he detected a similarity in their features, and the memory of the young man's blood puddling onto the pavement made Dr. Hoffman's own heart pause in fear. And yet it was the child's expression that held him. At night, when Alice had the lights turned low, the baby blinked and opened his eyes, and Dr. Hoffman thought he saw there a mute sympathy. Once he had stooped to put his lips to the child's head, an impulse less of kindness than of acknowledgment—though of what exactly, he could not have said.

He could not remember ever kissing a baby before.

But he had told Dr. Ludwig only that the child had been delivered directly to the nursery.

Now, at Alice's mention of the baby, he glanced toward the incubator that housed it, the last in a line of six. He felt a strange loneliness for a moment. Perhaps Alice's vague secretiveness was responsible, but it was Caro who came into his head. The few times he had seen her over the past several weeks, she had never repeated her request to tour the nursery, though he had not forgotten it. She came at night and sat in his garden with a copy of the *Tribune*. Roosevelt had called, in a radio address, for citizens to send him telegrams if they'd sign on to his remarkable National Industrial Recovery Act, and they were doing it, amazingly enough, in droves, flooding the telegraph companies. Caro approved of Roosevelt; she called him courageous. But more often she simply sat, staring into the dark and waiting for Dr. Hoffman. When they ate together —cold suppers left by the cook—they would talk, but more often he was too tired to eat, and they only went immediately to bed. She responded to him each time with the silent, ardent comfort of her own body offered to his.

She asked about the babies every day; she seemed to have

learned many of their names, just from hearing him talk about them. Sometimes, though, he was too discouraged to talk over the day's events, and he would put his hand over her mouth and pull her close to him. "I could never have survived this without you," he heard himself say one night.

"Tell me about little Helen," she had said, moving his hand away gently. "How is she today?"

"She is the same as yesterday, only an ounce bigger." In the dark next to him, he felt Caro smile.

"Which is the one that's blind? Bernice?"

Dr. Hoffman made a noise and rolled over to pin Caro beneath him. "Shhh. I don't want to talk about the babies. I see the babies in my sleep. Right now I only want to think about you."

She was quiet for a minute. Then she put up her hand and stroked his head. "Poor Leo," she said.

She smelled so good. She always smelled so good. He buried his face in her neck. He wanted to do something for her, to return the kindness of her affection.

But he could never think of anything to do.

Folding Helen's chart under his arm now, he walked over to the hatbox baby's incubator. The child's face, with its new weight, had begun to look less desperate.

You are becoming a beautiful baby, he thought, staring down at the baby's neat ear poking out from under its cotton cap, the curve of its cheek. *Will no one ever come to claim you?*

And then he thought of Caro again, the marvelous line of her throat as it fell into her breasts, the heart shape of her face in his hands, the sweetness of her skin.

He began to turn away slowly—he would be late for Dr. Ludwig. But something, some feeling, held him back a moment.

She had never said she wanted a baby. But she had wanted to see the nursery. He remembered that now with shame; he hadn't even thought about it these past few weeks. He had been so busy.

And yet now, now he could see himself placing the baby — this baby, this orphan baby — in Caro's arms. He could see the expression on her face. How he would love to be responsible for that much happiness! For it would make her happy; he felt sure of that. A wave of joy, unfamiliar and buoyant, rose in him. Could he give Caro a baby?

This baby, his baby who had come in a hatbox?

He turned back and regarded the infant one more time. *You have until the end of October,* he thought, watching the sleeping child's face. *You have just eight weeks, and then we shall all have to go home, wherever that is. Something needs to have been decided by then.*

And as he turned and left the nursery, he did not know whether he meant that as a warning to the baby's unknown mother, wherever she was, to come and fetch her child, or as a promise to himself.

Watching Dr. Hoffman go, Alice Vernon cradled close in her arms the baby Robert of the ruined face. She looked at the calm nursery around her, the cheerful wet nurses lined up in their rockers by the high window so that the light fell down on their heads, their talk full of the excitement of the morning, the elephants carrying away the prostrate Mrs. Taft and her cohorts. The walls of the nursery glowed in the early-afternoon sun; the tile floor gleamed. The incubators showed the bright reflections of the nurses passing back and forth in their white uniforms, the spirit traffic of angels hidden in the mirrored dimension of the glass doors. The order of the place pleased her, though she thought she saw it now in a new light.

Every day, she thought, rocking the baby, she could do this, at least. She could present to the forces of fate a readiness. She could offer comfort, warmth, light, milk. She looked down at Robert, at the pink slit that ran from his upper lip to the bottom of his nose, the red gum exposed beneath.

They got away this time, she thought, stroking the baby's head, *and they left their mark on you, though they did not finish you off. All we can do now is be watchful.*

Dr. Hoffman would not have condoned her role in what had happened this morning, but she saw that it had worked in all the ways she had hoped—Mrs. Taft and her friends had been routed, at least for the day, though she hoped for longer. The crowds had enjoyed the upset. And Dr. Hoffman, though perhaps he didn't even know it himself, had been cheered by the outward comedy of it. She could tell by the way he held himself now, by a relaxing of his neck and shoulders. She was glad to see it. The intensity of his efforts over the past few weeks had troubled her.

She would have to ask Louise to thank her friend, whoever he was.

Alice looked over at Louise now; she sat rocking with her friends, a baby at her breast. The night before, Louise had come into the nursery between feedings. Alice, who had been cleaning bottles, had been surprised to see her.

Louise had come over to where Alice stood at the sink and had begun idly turning the bottles on the drying rack.

"Don't do that." Alice glanced over at her. "You know not to touch those without washing your hands."

"Sorry." Louise put her hands away.

"Now I'll have to do them again." Alice removed the bottles, plunging them once again into the hot water.

"Sorry," Louise repeated. "I'll do them if you want."

Alice maintained a no-nonsense attitude with the wet nurses. They were good girls, but some of them were awfully young, and she had little tolerance for their troubles, which often struck her as immature and silly. They were good with their own babies—the camaraderie made the work of motherhood less onerous—but sometimes the girls were homesick and missed their husbands or boyfriends or, less often, their own mothers. Sometimes they had petty grievances with one another. Of the group at the fair this summer, Louise was a bit of a loner, less prone than the others to idle talk. Alice didn't consider her a troublemaker—there was nothing to fault her for, exactly—but the girl's confidences were so rare that Alice wondered what could have brought her into the nursery now.

"Alice," Louise began in a low voice. "I've heard something."

Alice plunged the brush into a bottle. She glanced over at Louise. The girl's tone—confessional and yet not pleading—made her take note.

"It's about those women, the ones writing letters in the newspaper." Louise reached out a hand toward the dripping bottles again but stopped herself in time. "What would you say if . . . what would you say if you knew that someone, a friend of ours, might have a way to stop them?"

Alice set the brush down. "What do you mean?" She had made no secret of her disdain for those opposing the incubator exhibit, but the way the girl spoke now suddenly made her regret having been so vocal about it.

"I have this friend—he's a friend of the whole nursery, really, though none of you know him. See, he was an early baby himself. He works here now, at the fair. He asked me—he told me—that the women were planning to picket the nursery tomorrow."

"He knows this?"

Louise shrugged. "He hears things, around the fair."

"I see." Alice picked up a soapy bottle, turned her attention to it again, trying to disguise her dismay. "Well, we've been waiting for that. I don't see that it's anything for you to worry—"

"He says he has a way of stopping them."

Alice stopped scrubbing and turned to face Louise. "What do you mean?"

"Oh, it's nothing *bad*!" Louise raised her eyebrows. "See, he has a plan. He knows everybody around here. He's friends with *lots* of the fair people. He says he can arrange . . . a disturbance."

Alice stared at her. The word *disturbance*—that was not Louise's word. "What do you mean? What kind of disturbance?"

"He didn't say exactly." Louise looked uncertain for a moment. She put her hands in the pockets of her dress. "But he says that people at the fair are mad about the letters. They don't like to see anyone at the fair criticized. They all have to stick together, he says." She looked away from Alice then, scanning the quiet nursery, the stationary rows of incubators.

Alice, following her gaze as if both could see suddenly beyond the shadowy room and out into the bright activity of the night streets, found herself becoming gradually aware of the presence of the fair around them—its hushed formal halls and galleries, its mesmerizing light shows, which trapped passersby on the broad avenues in a matrix of brilliant, trembling beams, the drone of airplanes crossing overhead, the authoritative voices over the loudspeakers, the displays of science and technology and knowledge. There was all that, Alice sensed, and then what lay behind it, too, the narrow streets filled with tumbling acrobats, the curbside inducements of midgets and Indians and snake charmers and magicians, the wild animals and carnival rides, the clowns on stilts stalking through the crowds, the painted women, and the apparition of figures from the past— the Little Dauphin, Abraham Lincoln, Joan of Arc, Paul Revere —mingling with ordinary fairgoers in a dark and thrilling conjunction of past and present.

"He wouldn't do anything dangerous, Alice," Louise said.

And with those words the balance between them had shifted, Alice sensed, Louise suddenly speaking to Alice as if from a vantage point of greater knowledge and authority, as if Alice were a child whose foolish protestations were born only of ignorance and fear.

"He means to help us," Louise said.

Alice had not known what to say. Yet she found, to her surprise, that she could trust Louise suddenly, Louise and her anonymous friend. She herself was no accomplice to these women insulting the nursery. If something happened to . . . throw them off course, well, then she would be glad of it. How easy it was, she discovered, to embrace this offer. "As long as no one is harmed," she said faintly.

"Will you tell Dr. Hoffman?"

Alice had thought a moment. Leo had gone to his rooms for the night. "It sounds as if . . . it sounds as if there is nothing one could do," she said, and though she was aware of the awkwardness of her phrasing, the obscurity of her answer, she did not dare venture further.

"I'll tell my friend then," Louise had said. "I'll tell him to go ahead."

And she had turned and left the nursery.

Alice rocked baby Robert for another few minutes, sitting quietly as the nurses milled around her, thinking of all that had happened that day, of all that had come to pass that summer. There were only a few weeks left before the fair would close and they could all go back to Coney Island. She would not be sorry to leave Chicago. It had been a sad, sorry summer, in many ways. She had enjoyed watching Mrs. Taft borne off this morning by that elephant and his majestic handler, but in a way it had frightened her, too.

She had spent most of her life now as a nurse. As thoughtless as death seemed to her, as cruel, it had a kind of strange authority and predictability to it. She could tell almost as well as Dr. Hoffman, she thought, when the end was near for a baby, and how it would happen. And then afterward you knew what had to be done. There were the things you did, always the same things, every time. She cried when the babies died, and even the sadness had a comforting sameness to it.

But now—now elephants could storm the streets and bear away your enemies. Now a stranger, a perfect stranger, could act on your behalf in such a grand and yet invisible way. Who was this man who could marshal the elephants? She felt herself —felt them all—in his debt somehow. And yet because she had never met him, never seen his face, she found she could imagine him capable of almost anything.

On the far side of the room, a nurse dropped a thermometer. The glass shattered with a far-off tinkling sound, and the room froze. Alice seemed to hear the sound over and over again, saw splinters of glass revolving in the air before bouncing slowly against the tile floor. She saw frost-colored beads of mercury race away to all four corners of the room, as if it were a polar field of invisible matter, the droplets drawn to the perimeter by magnets.

She would be glad when the summer was over, she thought, and a restlessness, almost an alarm, made her rise with difficulty to settle the baby Robert gently back in his incubator.

She observed that her knees had begun to hurt her when she sat for too long.

It has happened, she thought, *and I hardly noticed it until now.*

I'm getting old.

Evie had dressed carefully that morning, in a white blouse and a full dark gray skirt patterned with a snowfall of tiny white dots. She had paid a nickel to have her shoes shined.

"Hi, honey," Mr. Abbott had said to her when she'd stopped in to have a coffee before catching the elevated train. He called her honey for the color of her hair, he'd told her once. "The jars lined up on my mother's shelves," he said, "—they'd light up the whole room with sunshine. Just like you."

This morning he had set her coffee down on the counter with a paper napkin, half a banana, and a wink. She'd eaten the banana gratefully, put a dime under the saucer, and caught his eye at the grill to smile and wave at him when she left.

She had not told Sylvie where she was going. Sylvie had gotten a job with one of Balaban and Katz's movie houses, the Paradise on Crawford, and Evie scarcely saw her except on the rare evenings when she went to see a movie herself. Sylvie slept late in the mornings and came home long after the last show, when Evie had fallen asleep. Sylvie had dyed her hair a bright platinum, though she was, like Evie, a warmer blond by nature. She sat queenlike behind the ornate grille of the octagonal ticket booth at the front of the Paradise, painting her nails, eating sour balls she kept in a sack at her dimpled ankle, and smiling at the men and boys who came through. From her position at the end of the line, Evie would watch her sister grow larger and larger and brighter and brighter as the

line before the ticket booth dwindled, until at last she was facing Sylvie in her high glass box. Sylvie's expression, both imperious and mysterious at once, made Evie feel as if they were
strangers to each other. Sometimes their fingers met as Evie
pushed her money through the grille, and Sylvie, pushing back
a ticket, would lean forward and flash open her hand quickly,
palm down, as if flinging something away from her fingertips.
"Like my nails?" she would say. "Enjoy the show."

Evie went to see *King Kong*, squealing along with everyone
else at the massive mechanized ape and covering her eyes with
her hands, though it made her feel foolish to be so frightened.
She took two of her students, a pair of shy, red-haired brothers
a year apart, whom she sometimes saw playing on the street, to
see Walt Disney's *The Three Little Pigs*. On the way out they
waved to Sylvie. "That's my sister," Evie told the little boys.
They gaped.

In her high glass booth, filing her nails, Sylvie could be
mistress of all that took place in the wonderful, gilded theater.

But Evie also knew that Sylvie wept at night. The sisters
had moved in together after Jack's death, Sylvie taking up a
disorderly residence in their two small rooms. And sometimes
Evie lay awake on the daybed in the next room and listened
miserably to her sister's sobs.

"Don't talk to me," Sylvie had said the first time Evie had
gotten out of bed and tried to comfort her. "Just leave me
alone. I'll be all right."

But Evie could not forget the baby, either—the lost baby,
as she thought of him. She assumed that was why Sylvie cried.
That, and the loss of Jack.

"I can go and see," she offered one Sunday afternoon when
the sisters were having a meal together at the little table by the
window—bowls of soup and a plate of bread and cheese to

share, two golden pears so beautiful Evie almost hated to eat them. Evie knew that Sylvie hated Sundays; she said the church bells ringing all day were dreary. "I can just go and see if he's there, Sylvie," she repeated. "What can it hurt? Don't you want to know?"

Sylvie had said nothing at first. They had not spoken of the baby or of Jack since the night of Jack's death, beyond Sylvie's tacit acquiescence to the arrangements Evie had made for a modest service for Jack. Sylvie had been silent and withdrawn in the church that still, hot afternoon.

"What would it accomplish?" she said quietly at last, looking away from Evie. "Just going to see—what can you tell by seeing? I don't even know what . . . what it looked like."

Evie had been silent for a moment. "I would have to ask someone," she said finally. "Ask them if someone brought a baby in that day. A boy."

Sylvie looked out the window. Across the street, the door of the grocer banged. Two boys in short pants came running out and sped away down the empty sidewalk. A car turning the corner had to stop suddenly to avoid hitting them as they dashed across the intersection. "Things are different now," she said at last. "I don't want you going there. You promised me, anyway."

"But I think you would feel—"

"You promised me," Sylvie repeated. "It would only remind me of Jack all the time anyway."

Sylvie had risen from the table then and gone into the bedroom and closed the door. When she came out a few minutes later, Evie was still sitting at the table. Both sisters' eyes were red.

"I'm going out," Sylvie said. "Don't wait up."

Evie had spent the afternoon reading at the table by the window—Mr. Faulkner's new book *Light in August,* borrowed from the library; the principal at her school, a learned, quiet-

voiced man, too timid to be a good administrator, but a devoted
teacher, had recommended it to Evie. Transfixed, Evie read the
pages describing the pregnant woman's march across the coun-
tryside to find the man who would be her husband. At dusk
she closed the book and went out and took a walk, though the
heat was still oppressive and the smell in the street was foul.
She came back and got ready for bed when the sun began to
set, bringing a sandwich and *Light in August* to bed with her.
But all the while she was thinking of the baby, of finding him,
of the nurses' handing him to her—*We were hoping you'd come!
He's been waiting for you!*— and of him looking up into her
face and smiling.

And so on Monday morning, while Sylvie was still asleep,
Evie dressed in her polka-dot skirt and clean white blouse and
went out to break her promise.

She had been to the fair only in the company of
friends, and she felt daunted by the crowds. She bought a map
and sat down on a bench to unfold it. There were the tightly
wound streets of Paris—she found them with her fingertip.
There was the Lido, where the beautiful fan dancer Caro Day
performed. And there was the incubator exhibit building.

She stood up and began to walk. She did not know if she
was doing the right thing. She kept imagining that she saw
people she knew and felt embarrassed, realizing she could not
explain herself, doing this thing her sister had asked her not to
do. She knew that she had started to play a dangerous game
with herself, imagining herself holding the baby, giving the
baby a bottle, bathing the baby. But she couldn't help it. How
could Sylvie not want her own child? Surely if Evie were to
bring the baby home, Sylvie would change her mind.

She had stopped considering the fact that the infant might

have died, was in fact likely to have died. She could more easily imagine it lost in the world somehow, unnoticed in its hatbox, magically sustained, smiling up at her when she came
upon it and lifted the lid.

Four women with placards were marching back and forth in
a tight square in front of the steps of the building when Evie
came around the corner, her map in her hands. The storks, which
Evie had forgotten from her visit two months before, had retreated to the rear of the courtyard, where they shrank behind a
tree and picked at their feathers. The women were prosperous-
looking, with good jewelry and hats and white gloves, primly
hoisting their signs: ONLY ANIMALS BELONG IN THE ZOO!

Evie stopped. She had seen the letters in the newspaper and
read them carefully, mystified. Should she agree with them?
She liked to be right about things, and the letter writers
sounded so certain. But finding the women here today—
women sweating like ordinary people, the backs of their
dresses visibly wet—made her feelings clear to her. Didn't
these women know what went on inside? Hadn't they heard
how babies were rescued and saved and made well here, and
the parents never had to pay anything? She looked around as if
to summon help, for other people had stopped as well. They
hesitated on the sidewalk, staring impassively at the women
marchers, as if not wanting to commit themselves yet, one way
or the other. But Evie noticed that no line formed to go inside
for the noon showing, though it was only a few minutes before
twelve.

Could she simply walk past them? But the crowd around her
had grown already; now she would have to force her way through.
She glanced around. Three Indians in loincloths and feathers
and paint had appeared behind her. And behind them, a group
of talkative young women—ten or so—in bathing costumes

and shiny capes and diadems had settled themselves on the
wall by the courtyard, swinging their high heels and smoking
cigarettes. A scowling man with heavy black brows and a twirled
black mustache, wearing a riding habit and carrying a whip
coiled over his arm, passed suddenly in front of her, followed
by a tall, copper-haired woman in a blue sequined gown slit
daringly up her thigh.

Here was a group of ordinary-looking people—men in suit
trousers and white shirts and fedoras, women in sport frocks
and plain dresses and lace-up piqué summer hats—and beside them were three grimacing pirates. Here was a group of
children dressed all in blue—orphans?—and led by a ma-
tron; and here was a lady with a mustache, a man with a bird-
cage on his head, a woman in a Roman tunic. Four acrobats in
brilliant white sailor costumes and black shoes and white face
paint turned cartwheels in the street in front of her, scattering
children, and in the noisy, thickening crowd she saw clowns
—some in rainbow-colored wigs and turned-down mouths,
some in checkered pants and ruffles, some with huge false ears
pinned to wrinkled skullcaps—shouldering through the bystanders, waving tiny pistols and gibbering. Two more clowns,
fat as ticks in stuffed sequined suits, their painted mouths
smeared as though they had just eaten, sat down heavily on the
curb in front of her. When one leaned backward on a glittering
cane and wrenched open the front of his tunic, a dirty little
white dog with runny eyes hopped out and ran away barking,
returning a moment later with a large, half-smoked cigar held
in its teeth.

A Chinese dragon with palpitating flanks, brilliant in
shades of red and gold and orange, with huge, brimming black
eyes and a nodding head, undulated down the street, billowing
and bowing.

Somehow she lost her map. People were now overflowing the sidewalk and filling the street, but she noticed that most of them weren't watching the four protesters, who had slowed their pace and lowered their voices and were glancing nervously at the growing numbers of people around them. The crowd seemed simply to have been summoned to this point; people arrived and stayed, milling around and talking, lighting cigarettes, clapping one another on the back. She had to step back again to make room for a group of midgets—the men dressed in threadbare Victorian garb, the women in long gowns and ropes and chokers of pearls, feathered masks held to their faces. They came carrying tiny chairs and folding tables, with the legs sawed off halfway, which they set up on the sidewalk and proceeded to lay with a picnic of pickles and eggs and cheese and bread rolls.

"Almost time," said one of the midgets, leaning back and extracting from his vest a pocket watch.

And then someone shouted, "Here they come!" and Evie looked up to see four elephants proceeding down the street. A kind of bedlam broke out around her—people whistling and clapping and shouting and cheering. The women with the signs had stopped marching and were standing uncertainly, their signs drooping. The midgets had helped one another up to the top of their folding tables and were applauding seriously as if they occupied a reviewing stand.

And then it was over. The women had been borne away, screaming, and policemen spread out in the street like fishermen walking a net upstream, moving the chattering crowds along. Evie found herself swept up and carried along with the rest. Once she stopped and tried to turn back, but a policeman took her by the elbow. "Move along, miss. We've had quite enough excitement back there for one day. There's lots to see at the Century of Progress. Move along now."

And in that way she was led away from the incubator exhibit. Eventually the crowd dissipated enough for her to step
out of the stream of people and stop. The heat of the sun fell
like an anvil on her head. She moved toward the deep shade of
a wall opening into an alley, blinked as she entered the relative
darkness, and felt for the seat of the bench before her.

But another young woman was already sitting there. She
wore a white dress with a shawl collar, and a round blue hat,
which had slipped to the back of her head. Her hair was dark,
almost black, and coming loose from the bun at the nape of her
neck.

"Oh, you look like a nice person!" The woman leaned forward, crying out happily as if she had placed an advertisement
for such a position and was now gratified to have the candidate
appear, perfectly suited for the job. "I'm so glad you've come."

Evie blinked again. Was the woman speaking to her?

"Would you hold him for me?" The woman extended a
sleeping baby, blanket trailing. "Just for a minute—my husband's gone inside." She pointed to the building across the
street. THRILL HOUSE, read the letters on the front. Painted on a
mural over the entrance were six huge, frightening-looking,
cartoonish faces; each one was identified with a sign beneath
it: COKE ADDICT, KIDNAPPER, FIRE BUG, DRUG SLAVE, BOMBER, MANIAC.
"He's been inside for a long time, and I want to go and—" She
put the baby in Evie's arms; it felt warm and soft. "He's been in
there forever! I'll be right back. Promise!"

She darted away across the street, said something to the
ticket taker at the door—the words THRILL THEATER painted
overhead—and then disappeared.

Evie looked down at the baby in her arms. It had downy red
hair and pale, flawless cheeks, a bright strawberry mark on
one temple. The shadow of her own head moved over the

child's face as she bent to examine it. The baby grimaced suddenly and bunched itself up, but then it relaxed again, turning its head toward her shirtfront, keeping its eyes closed. It was heavy, and soft as bread dough; you wanted to tighten your arms around it. She bent down lower over the child and breathed in—delicious. And what a beautiful dress it had on, stitched at the collar with tiny blue xs—though she saw that the hem of the dress had unraveled in places, and the blanket was soiled at one corner.

Who would hand over their baby to a perfect stranger?

She looked up at the entrance to the Thrill House, but there was no one there now, not even the ticket taker. In fact, the little alley she had found herself in was deserted, and the sounds of the fair were far away, receding even as she strained to listen for them. She stood up quickly, the baby in her arms. Where was the mother? The baby turned against her, insistent; she looked down at it and saw then with perfect clarity a picture of herself in the future, a little red-haired boy on her lap, a book in front of them, their loving embrace. It was as if this image had been present before her always—a series of dots, particles of light she could not interpret until this moment.

She wanted a baby.

She sat back down, breathing hard, and then she stood up again. The child slept on heavily in her arms; she tried to hold it away from her body, stiffly, as if to disown it, but it was too heavy that way. Her arms began to ache. She wanted to put the baby down; it had become a dangerous thing, a temptation. But she could not just walk away and leave it. For one moment, then, she had a wonderful feeling of gratitude: the woman would never return; the baby would be hers to keep, and she would have rescued it.

No one came up or down the alley. Evie sat down again

finally, looked up at the sky as the minutes passed; she could see the sun moving bit by bit, the shadows against the far wall changing shape and density. The baby slept on in her arms. Evie felt her own eyes getting heavy. And then a bar of sunlight fell down the alley; Evie looked up, dazed, as the baby woke and began to cry.

The woman was hurrying toward her. "Sorry! Sorry! I couldn't find him anywhere! But he's coming now."

She reached down and scooped up the child. Evie looked up at her; she felt as if her face had been scalded.

"Do you want money?" The woman hoisted the baby in one arm and began to fumble in her purse with her free hand.

Evie stood up. "No. Please." She hurried away. She wanted to go home.

She would not tell Sylvie what had happened today.

ELEVEN

St. Louis poled the black gondola through the still, warm waters of the lagoon. "I could do *this*," he suggested to Caro, who was lying in the darkness at the other end of the boat, leaning back against a pillow, her hands behind her head.

"Look, a star." She pointed over St. Louis's head into the clouds of the night sky, which were thick as black batter and oppressively low.

St. Louis didn't look up. The gondola was more awkward to steer than he'd anticipated. He poled faster, trying to avoid the fabricated mossy bank of the Enchanted Island, which had loomed up suddenly in the darkness. A section of the half-buried chicken wire that contained the sloping shore of the island flashed at him in the dark as they glided past. For a moment he thought of ice, and an image of the fairgrounds as they would be in winter came into his head—a cold surf of snow blowing across the wide avenues and banked in glassy layers against the monuments, filaments of ice strung from the

Havoline thermometer and the frozen cable cars and silent Temple of Jehol. How still and cold and colorless it would be then. How unthinkably empty.

"Two stars." Caro spoke again from the other end of the boat. Her arm floated up again, pointing.

She wasn't paying attention. St. Louis reached up to mop his forehead; even at night this week the fairgrounds were stifling. He'd read in the *Tribune* that morning how a man had died, sleepwalking off the roof of his apartment building. The account in the paper reported that the man had told a neighbor he was going to drag his bed up to the roof for relief from the unnatural heat and to catch the night breeze, if there was any to be caught. St. Louis had pictured the man, the line of his fatal descent to the street. But he did not want to think of the unfortunate sleeper now.

"Of course, it would be better in Venice," he said, trying to reel Caro in, draw her attention.

Caro raised herself to her elbows. "What would?"

"Being a gondolier."

She lay back down again. "Wouldn't anything be better in Venice?"

"How would you know?"

"That's what they say."

The gondola tipped suddenly. St. Louis dropped to a crouch and grabbed at the side. Caro laughed quietly.

"Maybe they're too tippy." St. Louis rose cautiously to his feet and resumed poling. It was the first time he'd had Caro alone to himself in what felt like weeks, and he wanted just to keep talking, to keep her there; he did not want to think of the heat, or men stepping off rooftops, their eyes closed, dangerous dreams skating across the fields of sleep. It was clear to him that Caro had taken a lover—how else to account for her disappearances at night, her new, quiet face?—but he didn't know who it was, and he was too proud to follow her and try to find out, even though he was tempted.

But he was so glad to see her tonight. He'd come into her dressing room a little past midnight after her last show and put his hands over her eyes, even though she could see him perfectly well and had given him a welcoming smile in her mirror from beneath the nodding feathers of her headpiece.

"Guess who?" he said.

Caro frowned, pretending to think. "Lionel Barrymore?"

"Nope."

"Jimmy Cagney?"

"No."

"Ramon Novarro?"

"No, no, no." He'd dropped his hands. "Caro," he'd said, meeting her eyes in the mirror. He hadn't even tried to disguise the pleading in his voice. "Come on. I haven't seen you for weeks. Come and take a gondola ride with me. Please."

"You don't know how to steer one of those," she'd said. "And you're not supposed to take them at night anyway." But she had come with him all the same.

He was full of the day's triumph, full of wanting to talk. The escapade with Mrs. Taft and her friends had cost him four hundred dollars, a hundred for each of the elephant's trainers, but he considered it worth every penny. He would not forget anytime soon the sight of those women being evacuated, as he liked to term it to himself, from in front of the baby house. He'd thought of everything, even paying off the cops, who might have made trouble for the elephant handlers. Best of all, though, he could do it whenever the occasion arose— maybe not the elephants again, but something else, surely, would come to him? For the occasion *was* sure to arise again.

He did not expect Mrs. Taft to give up easily. Her face, when he had drawn close once that morning before she was scooped up by the elephant, was severe and bloodless; he'd had the impression she might be balding under the grim thatch of a hairpiece that had been knocked askew in her ascent to the elephant's back.

Meanwhile, though, he had inadvertently discovered a wonderful source of information about Mrs. Taft's intentions: the chatty bartender employed by the fair's trustees to pour libations at their meetings. The fair board members lunched together weekly in a heavily curtained room at the Drake. St. Louis had met the bartender playing cards at the Café de la Paix one night and in a short time had discovered the man's occupation. After that, it was simple—St. Louis put him on a generous retainer, and the man passed on anything he thought St. Louis might find interesting. When he'd overheard a heated argument among several of the trustees, including Mr. Taft, about Mrs. Taft's proposed protest at the incubator exhibit, he'd stopped by the fair that evening and left a note for St. Louis with Trudi, the hostess.

St. Louis had been gratified by the alacrity of the fair people's responses to his plea for help. All day, after the event had been pulled off successfully, people stopped him to shake his hand or clap him on the shoulder.

Even Dr. Anton Oleksak, the ancient chess champion who would play blindfolded anyone willing to spend a dollar and risk looking the fool, had paused over arranging his pawns when St. Louis sat down opposite him late that afternoon on the shady sidewalk near the planetarium, where Anton had set up shop for the day.

"Prepare to die," St. Louis had said, pulling out the rickety bamboo chair Anton supplied and rolling up his sleeves. It was what he always said; but he'd never beaten Anton, though he'd played him two or three times a week all summer, whenever he ran across him.

But Anton had lifted up a corner of his blindfold and grinned at St. Louis through his wrinkles and his long, wispy, sand-colored beard. "Ah! It is the famous short man, St. Louis Percy," he said, "local hero."

It seemed the day's adventure had given him a kind of in-house celebrity. That afternoon, he'd taken a seat at Walgreens on one of the counter's one hundred green-topped stools, which stretched away like a forest of neat little shrubs, and the boy behind the counter had instantly brought him a towering banana split. "On the house," the boy said, putting down the silver dish in front of St. Louis, who'd planned on having only coffee. "My boss says you deserve it." The boy handed him a newspaper, folded to the comics—*Moon Mullins, Winnie Winkle the Breadwinner, Dick Tracy, Gasoline Alley*. "Want a paper, mister? Shoe shine?"

At the Horticulture Building, a pretty, smiling young woman, wearing one of the season's wide cartwheel hats and dipping here and there among visitors with a tray full of pamphlets and blossoms, had pinned a peony to his shirt—pure white threaded with deep cerise—and kissed him on the cheek.

Even the notoriously ill tempered Madame Boulanger, proprietress of the popular trained-dog act, had stood up from feeding her four slavering white French bulldogs—Moselle, Yvonne, Colette, and Beau Geste, whose cavelike mouths dripped rusty lengths of drool—and threw him a salute from beneath the bandstand risers where she had set out the dogs' bowls in the shade. The spots of rouge on her cheeks glowed like coals in the heat of the day.

Everywhere he went, people congratulated him.

But Caro hadn't said anything yet.

"So," he began, working the pole carefully through the water, "aren't you going to congratulate me?"

"What for?"

St. Louis looked down the length of the gondola. "What *for*? You didn't see my little diversion today?"

Caro sat up, as if alerted by something in St. Louis's voice. "What diversion?"

"My"—St. Louis didn't know what to call it, exactly —"my *fait accompli.*"

Caro stared at him. He could see the pale oval of her face through the dark.

"What are you talking about?" she said.

"At the *baby* house. The women . . . the *elephants.*" He was incredulous. "Didn't you even *hear* about it?"

There was a silence. Then Caro said, "You arranged that?"

St. Louis blew on his fingertips—the gesture of a man on a winning streak. "I have taken a real liking to those babies," he said. "You remember, they and I have something in common?" But as soon as he said it, he was sorry. He knew his tone was absurd and pompous. It wasn't what he'd meant to say. He'd thought she would enjoy the story, be delighted by it, that it would awaken in her some of their old complicity. But she was being so serious. She'd always had a serious side; even her dancing, he thought, had a serious side. It was the combination that made her show more than just another skin opera— the frank suggestion of sex mixed with a sensuous gravity that just approached something unspeakable and private in her nature and then veered away before too much had been revealed. It wasn't that she thought what she did was art—she didn't mistake it for art, he thought. But she knew how good she was, and she didn't underestimate her effect. She took it seriously, and that allowed the men who so loved her to take it seriously, too, to fall completely under her spell. Men fell in love with Caro's own brand of almost helpless seduction.

That she might be a prisoner to it had never occurred to him before, but as he looked at her now he found himself wondering again about who her lover might be and, for the first time, whether there was a chance she might be hurt by this new affair. He'd had to discourage plenty of Caro's castoffs over the years. Yet somehow he didn't think this engagement—whoever it was with—would end that way. She'd been too close-mouthed about it for it not to matter.

"I've been thinking," he hurried on. "I might want to be a doctor."

The words, reprehensible things, flew out of his mouth and hung there in the air between him and Caro. He hadn't meant to say them! He hadn't even known he even felt such a thing! He'd only intended to make her laugh. But now that the words were said, and in that awful, flat, truthful way, like a statement of confession, he realized that he *had* imagined it. It was pure fantasy—ridiculous!—himself a doctor like Hoffman, saving babies. He drove the pole deep down into the mud at the bottom of the lagoon and pushed off violently. He was to be pitied. She would pity him for entertaining such a foolish notion. He pitied himself.

"In my spare time, of course," he added then, hoping to make it better, but it came out with such bitterness that he surprised even himself. He gave up. He sat down at his end of the gondola and looked away from Caro toward the shore.

"Doctors don't have much spare time."

He turned to look at her, but she was sitting up now, hugging her knees, and gazing away toward the shore. "What do you want, St. Louis?" she said abruptly. "You don't want *money*.

But maybe you want to buy a house someplace. Maybe you want to go home?"

She had turned to look at him. He felt her eyes on his profile.

"You're miserable," she went on. "Every time you open a newspaper, you're looking for work. You don't *need* work; we both know that. But you're not happy anymore. You haven't been happy all summer. It's been building and building. What can I do?"

How like her this was. Just when he despaired of ever being able to reach her again, she showed him she had been watching the whole time. In school, when they were young, there had been a time when St. Louis had been the victim of unkindness at the hands of some older boys: They'd called him Toad and sat on him and dribbled spit onto his cheek and told him the girls wanted to kiss him; and then one fall day at recess they dragged a girl over, a skinny, olive-skinned girl with brown hair and thin shins lashed with a summer's worth of welts and scratches, who screamed when she was made to kneel down next to St. Louis and kiss him. He had shut his eyes tightly so as not to see the look on her face. "I'm sorry," he'd said to the hot dust of the ground. "I'm sorry."

Caro didn't say anything to him about this incident at first —he wasn't sure she'd even known about it—but a few days later, the brown-haired girl had crossed the street in town to come up to him as he stood holding his uncle Warren's team of horses. "They shouldn't have done that to you," the girl said bluntly, standing before him and balancing curiously on one foot. "To us. Your cousin says they will go to hell for it and rot forever, and their eyes will fall out, and rats will eat their fingers." She waited, looking at him, and then shifted to the other foot and sighed. "I shouldn't have yelled so much when they made me kiss you," she said. "You're not so bad. Anyway, *I* won't go to hell. I think you're a nice boy."

St. Louis had reddened, and she had walked away, hopping from one foot to the other, obviously relieved. A few days later at school, he saw her staring adoringly at Caro, polishing an apple on her dress and offering it up.

At the time, it was Caro's indirectness in the matter of his defense that he had admired. And then, a day or so later, after school one afternoon, Caro had beaten up one of the biggest, meanest boys, the one St. Louis considered his personal tormentor. She had blackened the boy's eye and scraped his face on the ground until it bled.

"I wanted to wait," she told St. Louis that night at home. They sat on the porch, leaping down from the steps from time to time to cup the last fireflies of the season, enjoying the greenish glow inside their laced fingers. "I wanted to wait until he wasn't expecting me to come after him anymore. That way I scared him, too. Now he'll be scared of me forever." She had thrown open her hand; a spray of bottle-green sparks flew out and away.

St. Louis had thought his admiration could know no bounds.

"Caro," he began now. "Caro." He wanted to make up something, something that would distract her—distract him—from what had begun to feel like the inevitable truth. He saw that as much as he could not stand the thought of being parted from her, she could not bear the thought of losing him, either. And yet it would probably happen anyway.

This time, though, he decided not to lie.

"I don't know," he told her. "I don't know what you can do."

The gondola drifted. Caro sat far away at the other end, waiting, obscure in the darkness. They could have been anywhere, he thought suddenly, staring around at the heavy black skirt shapes of the willow trees that enveloped the shores of the la-

goon. The lights of the fair were turned off; far away was a twinkling wall of light that was Michigan Avenue, a distant iceberg,
glittering.

"Let me know when you figure it out," she said.

But there was no irony in her voice.

"All right. What does he want?" Alice Vernon turned
around and faced Louise. She felt unnerved, and she knew her
voice betrayed her. Yet there was no good reason for it, was
there? After all, what could this friend of Louise's possibly
want that she would not freely give him, if she could? Alice
would not soon forget the sight of Mrs. Taft, sign flapping,
being borne away on the back of the elephant. She thought it
one of the greater satisfactions of her life. And now Louise had
promised that this "friend" would always "take care of" such
matters, though Alice did not see how he could guarantee such
a thing. Had he some special dispensation that allowed him
to read the future, predict the next attack—should there be
another—against the nursery? Still, she was aware of having
been done a favor by this stranger, and aware that Dr. Hoffman
knew nothing of her complicity in the matter.

"Alice!" Louise protested. "You make it sound so awful!"

They were standing in the small, windowless kitchen annex
that served the nursery's purposes—hearty breakfasts and
heavy lunches at a plain, round refectory-style table, prepared
by an unwilling and morose cook who seemed to speak very
little English. The cook served dinner four nights a week; the
other three, the girls were given an allowance to eat at the fair.
Sometimes, one of the wet nurses took it upon herself to cook
for the others, usually something she herself was homesick for,
fried chicken or spaghetti or pierogi, things that required making what Alice referred to as an ungodly mess.

Alice leaned back against the sink now and put her hands on the cold enamel. Through the glass door that led out to a short flight of steps, she could see waves of heat shimmering against the white wall of the next building, a squat souvenir shop in the shape of the Arc de Triomphe, where people bought jaunty black berets or miniature gold-painted Eiffel Towers, their bases packed with sand, the words CENTURY OF PROGRESS printed on tiny red, white, and blue felt flags that flew from the tops of the towers.

She smothered a feeling of impatience, returned her hands to the front of her uniform and clasped them together. What was it about Louise that made her distrust the girl? It was that she was stupid, Alice concluded, though pronouncing this sentence on Louise made her feel old and ill-natured. There was nothing in the credentials for a wet nurse that said she had to be clever, after all, only kind and healthy and not too preoccupied with her own needs, but Alice suspected Louise of overestimating her own ability to think things through in an intelligent manner. Louise, Alice suspected, might bite off more than she could chew.

Louise laughed. Alice felt the back of her neck flush and begin to itch.

But hurriedly, as if sensing the climate of Alice's mood, Louise said, "He only wants the simplest thing. The sweetest thing, really. And he didn't even say it at *all* like we owed it to him. He wants—" Louise took a breath. "He wants to come and hold a baby sometime."

"What?" Alice's tone conveyed shock. And yet it was partly manufactured—she'd had a feeling about this, hadn't she?

"It's not so strange, Alice," Louise went on. She pulled out a chair and sat down, as if to reduce her size in front of Alice. "Don't act like it is. There are lots of people who come to the hospital back home—the rockers, you call them, right? I've seen them. Mother even came for a while, remember? And you've said yourself it's good for the babies to have people holding them and loving them. Honestly, he's the nicest man." Louise paused for a minute. "I think he's lonely, in a way. He hasn't any children of his own—"

"We are not here to comfort the lonely, Louise—"Alice began in a high tone.

But Louise did not let her finish. "He was born premature himself." She looked up at Alice. "He thinks it may account for him looking the way he does."

"How *does* he look?" Alice's tone sounded absurdly alarmed, even to herself.

Louise sighed. "Oh, well, he's short. Not like a midget exactly, but almost. And he's got bad eyes. And he's ugly, but in a kind of nice way."

"Ugly in a nice way," Alice said dryly. "I see."

Louise stood up, impatient. "You don't have to do anything for him. He didn't even ask. He's just talked about it so often, and I thought I'd ask you. He's a real friend to us, Alice. You've no idea."

Alice looked at Louise's face. There was no guile there. Alice thought herself a good judge of guile. She considered. There were only a few weeks left of the fair. She did not want Dr. Hoffman upset, and more demonstrations would surely worry him. He had been so distracted, sorry about the babies who had died, of course, and doing his job assiduously as always, even heroically. She knew he was exhausted. But there was something else troubling him, she felt sure. Perhaps he *would* close the hospital after this summer, take up Dr. Ludwig's offer to join his staff at Sarah Morris. Once, she had thought Dr. Hoffman would never be tempted by such a thing, but this summer had been so arduous—so hot, she thought now, so *disturbed.* And if Dr. Hoffman went, she would have to go, too. No longer would she be free to run her own nursery—for she considered herself Dr. Hoffman's partner in some ways, though not his equal.

She watched Louise, who stared back at her stubbornly.

"All right," she said at last. "I will let you know a good time for him to come." She pushed away from the sink and began to leave. A feeling of embarrassment had come up in her, as though she and Louise had made some arrangement of which Alice ought to be ashamed.

She turned back. "What is your friend's name?" she began, with an effort at courtesy.

Louise smiled. "St. Louis," she said. "For the city, not the saint!" She waggled a finger at Alice. "That's how he always says it."

"I see." Alice moved toward the door. "Well, I will find a good time, and then your St. Louis may come and rock the babies. But just once—I am only promising once."

"You'll see," Louise said. "You'll see."

Still, St. Louis was not what she had expected.

Alice picked a night when Dr. Hoffman was out to dinner with Dr. Ludwig. This, too, gave her a feeling of being dishonest with him, but she could not very well explain it to him now, and there would only be the one occasion, as she saw it.

It was, first, that he brought flowers. He came staggering in under an armload of white roses—"left over from the Hawaiian Day festivities," he explained easily. "There were pineapples, too, but I couldn't carry as many of those, and I liked the roses better. Shame to waste them." He put them into Alice's arms as if it were the most natural thing in the world. Alice, to whom no

one had ever given roses, was overcome by their weight and
scent. "I am your servant, madam," he said to her, bowing low.
"I wish a place like this had been around when I was born."
And then he looked over the nursery with what Alice could see
instantly was clear and respectful admiration.

"I want you to know," he said, turning back to her, "that I was
glad to do what I did." He brought it out in the open like that,
right away, as if he were not accustomed to making or keeping
secrets. Alice found herself relaxing. "She's an awful woman,
and the things she said in the newspaper were criminal. But
you don't owe me anything for the trouble, Miss Vernon. I'd do it
again, just to keep people like her where they belong. It's un-
conscionable, what they'll print in the newspapers these days."

My, she thought. *And well spoken, too. But not* too *well spoken.*

It was, also, that he was ugly, and yet his ugliness did not offend, as Louise had said. He had the features of a dwarf, Alice
recognized—the heavy forehead and eyes set deep into his
face—and yet his face had humor and intelligence and kindness. He was not so short as most dwarves she had seen; there
were colonies of them on Coney Island, where they worked at
the amusement park. They walked along the sidewalks as if
they occupied a different stratum than other people, which she
supposed they did, in a way, most things being out of reach for
them. But there was nothing watchful or downtrodden about
St. Louis's face, Alice concluded, searching for a gown for him
to wear. Nothing anxious. His hair was a soft chestnut color,
warm and gleaming as a child's. There was an athletic vigor to
his body, but it was not a coiled or threatening strength. More
an optimistic sort of energy.

Before long he was scrubbed and gowned. He looked rather
comic in the long sleeves and trailing hem, but he did not
seem to recognize this, standing still and serious for Alice as

she tied the strings for him in back, holding his arms out straight so that the sleeves dipped like angels' wings. And then she led him to a rocking chair and put a baby in his lap. She picked Robert, despite or maybe because of his ruined face. And as she settled Robert in St. Louis's arms, he looked down at the baby and then up into her face and then down at the baby again with an expression of such joy—*The privilege of this,* his face seemed to say, *the extraordinary privilege of it*— that Alice felt her heart contract.

"Well," St. Louis said, taking a deep breath, looking down into Robert's face. "Well. OK. Hi there."

And then he glanced up at Alice again. "I've never held a baby before," he said fiercely, and she was touched.

"It doesn't hurt him?" he asked her when she came back a few minutes later. He was staring down at Robert. "His lip being like that?"

"No." She watched his face for signs of disgust, but he showed none.

He didn't say anything else then. He just rocked steadily, holding Robert carefully, giving the baby a kind of rapt attention. Once Alice came over and smiled down at St. Louis. "If he's uncomfortable, he'll let you know," she told St. Louis. "You don't have to watch him all the time as if he's going to explode. You could even close your own eyes and relax. We do, sometimes."

St. Louis looked up at her. "I might miss something," he said.

And so after that Alice left him alone. She found she almost forgot about him. It was her favorite time of day, the first evening shift. The public showings were over until the next day; the wet nurses were sleepy themselves. Over the course of the summer in Chicago, as the babies had gained weight—those that had survived—they had become stronger and had also grown accustomed to Alice's regimen of day and night; many slept their longest stretches at night now, and though Alice woke them for feedings, those feedings, in the dim light, seemed calmer, quieter. Babies nursed peacefully and went back to sleep.

But then all at once there were four babies crying suddenly —often after feedings there were infants in distress from the effort required by immature stomachs for digestion. She took one baby in her arms, and Nan took another; a wet nurse who had stayed after the others, to finish with an especially small infant too weak and sleepy to nurse efficiently, accepted a third— and then Alice caught herself looking over at St. Louis. And when she took Robert, who was sleeping peacefully, away from him and put the second baby in his arms instead, a scowling, bawling boy of just over four pounds now, nearly large enough to go to the Home for the Friendless if his mother never came back for him, she saw how St. Louis reached up with not a single sign of fatigue or distress, despite having been sitting there for nearly two hours, and when the child was held against St. Louis's chest, it gave a whimper and then quieted, its mouth open, blowing a sweet breath on St. Louis's chin. It was funny, Alice thought—in St. Louis's arms, the baby did not look so small.

And then she saw with surprise that St. Louis was crying— a sliding curtain of wet ran from his eyes and washed over his cheeks.

What was it? she thought. What was it that moved him so now? "Are you tired?" she whispered.

But he shook his head no.

She smiled down at him. "You're a natural," she said in a whisper, and patted his shoulder.

And as she walked away back to her own charge, she thought, *He's like Dr. Hoffman.*

He has the touch.

St. Louis had not approached the hatbox baby. He had not even seen him. He had almost forgotten about him, in fact, though he had meant to find a way to ask about him or at least lay eyes on him. He had expected to be interested in what went on in the nursery, expected to come away with information —how they did this or how they did that, whatever they did, however they secured the future for these helpless creatures who depended so utterly on the care and skill and intelligence of these adults.

But instead he had found himself completely absorbed by the children in his arms—first Robert, with his face that looked as if a sharp hoof had stamped angrily on the baby's tender bow of a mouth, and then Samuel, against whose warm, smooth cheek he had dared to rest his own for a moment before giving him up. It had made him think about his own mother again, to sit there like that, and he had not thought about her in years and years. Holding the babies, he had envisioned himself being held, how his mother must have held him, and the imagined impression of her body against his own had made him feel weak with grief. And yet he could not fully make the leap that would allow him to remember himself as a baby, and so in his musings he had been able to imagine himself being held only by *himself;* he had been split in two, divided between his past and his present, both caretaker and dependent, adult and infant, equally a memory and an irrefutable, immediate presence for whom the act of sheltering another human being in his arms had occasioned a violent and yet ecstatic awakening.

Alice had come to take Samuel away at last. She had been in a hurry, worried about something, he had sensed. And then he had realized that Hoffman had not been at the nursery all night, and that Alice obviously had not told Hoffman of St. Louis's arranged presence there that evening. Perhaps he was expected back soon. And Hoffman likely did not know of St. Louis's role with the elephants, either, he decided, handing Alice his gown and bidding her good night. He had wanted Alice to be grateful to him for his alacrity in leaving, because he was grateful to her for what he now thought of as a transforming moment in his life.

He had envied Hoffman before; here was a man with the best sort of authority, the authority to do good, the only sort St. Louis thought he could recognize and respect anymore. But now he felt a strange and surprising affinity with Hoffman. He had sat where Hoffman himself sometimes sat. He had held babies whom Hoffman had held and touched and examined. And he had felt something, something passing between those babies and himself. At the exhibit of the Massachusetts Institute of Technology, he had stood once in an expectant, silent crowd and watched the spectacle of a million-volt current leaping a three-foot gap between poles. *That* was what had gone between him and those babies.

Thomas Edison—at least, he *thought* it was Edison—had been asked once what electricity *was*.

"I don't know," Edison had reportedly said. "Nobody knows. Sometimes—I think—it's God."

But Hoffman knew the *feeling* of electricity, St. Louis thought, the feeling that a brilliant cable—a leaping, flying beam of light thrown from one canyon edge to another—now tied you to another human being.

Hoffman knew that feeling, St. Louis thought. He *must*.

And now St. Louis knew it, too.

TWELVE

St. Louis had arranged for Sully to work the end of Caro's last show that evening; he hadn't known how long he might be at the baby house. Leaving the nursery, he discovered he was ravenous with a kind of appetite he hadn't had in weeks. He went to the Café de la Paix and sat in the kitchen amid the confusion and chaos of the evening's last dinner orders. He liked a busy kitchen—that was something else he'd missed all these years, he thought, the simple, domestic pleasure of a kitchen. Things he'd missed seemed to be stacking up fast around him: a permanent home, a warm kitchen. A baby. He did not let himself think of a wife. He had not ever let himself think about a wife.

In the Café de la Paix, waiters stopped by the table in the back between orders to listen to a replay of the Cubs game on the radio—Charlie Root had pitched a no-hitter against the Pirates at Wrigley Field. St. Louis ate two bowls of French onion soup, sopping up the last of the broth with the leftover ends of the loaves of bread, and then Trudi brought him an untouched chocolate mousse, grown warm and pooling on the plate, and a glass of almost flat champagne. He held a private celebration over his meal, passing out cigars to the waiters and cooks and dishwashers. He'd enjoyed washing dishes this summer, he thought, and noted the nostalgia of his feeling. Yet it did seem as if it were over now, somehow. Or nearly over, anyway.

But he'd liked standing at the sink, listening to the ball game. Once, he'd caught the "prairie poet" Carl Sandburg reading his verses over the air. St. Louis liked poetry. He liked that strange poem a bartender in New York had shown him once, "A Song for Occupations," by that fellow Walt Whitman. It was mostly a list of tools and trades, but St. Louis, who appreciated the art of physical labor, thought it had a kind of grandeur to it. He could still recite parts of it:

> The calking-iron, the kettle of boiling vault-cement, and
>   the fire under the kettle,
> The cotton-bale, the stevedore's hook, the saw and buck of
>   the sawyer, the mould of the moulder, the working-knife
>   of the butcher, the ice-saw, and all the work with ice,
> The work and tools of the rigger, grappler, sail-maker,
>   block-maker,
> Goods of gutta-percha . . .

Once he'd known a whole lot of it.

Waiters came in one by one and shed their white aprons while he sat at the table. The last patron finally left. Fred Waring's radio orchestra, the Pennsylvanians, came on. The waiters took seats around St. Louis, talking over the night and counting tips and downing glasses of ice water and accepting plates of leftover chops and broiled tomatoes, the tomatoes cooled now and fallen in on themselves.

The baseball game ended, the news came on. Nazi storm

troopers had attacked Catholics visiting Munich on a church convention for wearing orange shirts, an offense against the brown Nazi uniform; everyone seated at the round table in the Café de la Paix shook their heads over the Nazis.

Hitler and Il Duce, someone said—what a pair.

The Prince of Wales had turned thirty-nine in June but was still receiving birthday gifts. Mahatma Gandhi was beginning another death fast. Kurdish fighters in Iraq had massacred eight hundred Assyrians.

St. Louis leaned forward to knock the tip of ash on his cigar into a ceramic ashtray fashioned to look like the face of a Polynesian parrot; he would miss these people, he thought suddenly, looking around at their faces. Together they listened quietly for another minute: the playwright Winchell Smith, author of *Brewster's Millions* and *Lightnin'*, had died at the age of sixty-two. Bad boy Elliott Roosevelt, the president's playboy son, had divorced his second wife in Nevada. Roosevelt himself was resting at Hyde Park . . .

At last, St. Louis stood up and patted the shoulder of the young waiter beside him, who was bent over, eating furiously. Maybe he didn't get enough at home. What was his name?

"Johnny, right?" St. Louis said.

The young man looked up gratefully. He had a big nose, crushed like an oyster shell; probably an amateur boxer, St. Louis thought, recognizing the injury.

"So long, chief," the kid said, happy.

"So long."

"Good night," they called as he went out the back door.

He stopped in the alley by his hammock, but he wasn't feeling tired. He checked his pocket watch. It was only half past midnight—he might catch Caro before she left the Lido for the night. He hadn't told her about going over to see the babies;

she'd been meeting with a costumer and a hat designer when he'd stopped by the Lido in the late afternoon, and he hadn't had a chance to go back. But he wanted to tell Caro about the babies now. Maybe she'd even come to one of the showings with him tomorrow. He could point out to her the babies he'd held.

He walked down the alley and stepped into the street. There were plenty of people out still, couples mostly. In the moonlight, and under the chalky glow of the streetlights, the women in their silvery chiffon stockings and white doeskin gloves and white walking sticks looked like pale moths. Something about the light from the streetlights sapped the color from the scene before him: the shiny mirrors of wet tables and the empty scrollback chairs at the cafés, the long batons of furled awnings, the cobblestones stretching away in a shallow black river. The men seemed bodiless and insubstantial beneath the billow of their white shirts.

Once again St. Louis felt a shivery premonition of winter. Time sped past, the season of heat and invention replaced by the tragic and glacierlike face of December, January, February; he hadn't meant to conjure it up for himself, but there the image was anyway: a host of startled, frozen pedestrians, the women hopeful, eternally poised in their white summer frocks, the men with their white sleeves outstretched protectively, all of them indistinct and colorless and anonymous under a thick shell of ice, stalled through the winter's long night.

When a white-haired waiter leaned over a railing suddenly and dashed the ice from a champagne bucket across the street at St. Louis's feet, the tumble of flashing blocks broke over his shoes with the sound of glass shattering.

"Sorry, pal." The old waiter, his bucket raining drops as he backed away, apologized with a series of rapid, obsequious bows in St. Louis's direction.

Caro was not in her dressing room. Sully, who was sweeping sawdust down the dimly lit hall backstage, said he'd escorted her home and then come back to clean up.

St. Louis went back out into the street. Sometimes, standing on the steps of the Lido, especially at night, and in the dark like this, he thought about the boy who had been killed, about what had happened to him here—at St. Louis's own threshold, as it were. But tonight he wanted to catch Caro before she left again to meet whoever it was she'd been meeting, or before she turned out her light, should this be one of the rare evenings she decided to stay in.

He began to walk in the direction of Caro's apartment above the store. But turning into one of the fair's alleys, he realized that he must be coming up behind the baby house; he had never come this way before. The passage was not more than ten feet wide, banked on one side by the slick wall of the Arc de Triomphe souvenir shop, and by a stone wall on the other. St. Louis was pleased to put up his hand and encounter real stone; one longed for the warmth of such materials in this cool landscape of copper and glass, chromium and steel.

A flutter in the branches of the tree over his head—a mimosa, he thought in surprise, holding out his hand and catching a drifting, feathery blossom on his palm—made him look up. Something was up there; he could hear it moving about, invisible in the darkness. It wasn't a bird, though, he thought. It sounded too big for that.

And then he saw the monkey—Capuchin, the organ-grinder's monkey. It swung down toward him suddenly on one long arm, like a weight falling down a string, and then swooped back up into the branches. St. Louis stepped back a few paces, but he couldn't see the creature in the darkness. He approached the tree and put his hand against the trunk; he heard the monkey ascend higher into the branches. What was it doing up *there*? he wondered. Where was the old organ-grinder?

It was easy enough to climb up into the tree. Maybe if he sat quietly in the branches, the monkey would come and climb into his lap and he could carry it back where it belonged. He'd seen the monkey do that with the organ-grinder, folding itself up against the old man's soiled shirt. St. Louis had thought it childlike, the way it stared out at people from its safe haven with bulging, round black eyes. The organ-grinder was a drinker, one of those men ruined by the cheap liquor that circulated during Prohibition; St. Louis had played cards with him, too, though the old man preferred to play with the animal trainers and handlers and stable boys out in the sweet-smelling barns near the water. St. Louis had seen him only once or twice at the Café de la Paix's nightly game.

When he was sitting on the branch near the top of the stone wall, he rested a moment. He had not climbed a tree in a long time; it had been harder work than he remembered. He peered up into the darkness of the branches. He could see Capuchin, sitting several limbs above him, holding on to the trunk of the tree with one arm, and with the other, flicking its tail back and forth nervously across its white face. Well, he would have to wait for the creature to settle down.

And then he looked over the stone wall.

He was looking down into a small, shadowy paved courtyard, furnished with a black wrought iron table and a pair of chairs. Several large enameled pots planted with flowering shrubs glowed in the darkness. The only entrances to the courtyard were an arched gate in the wall below where St. Louis sat in the tree and a set of French doors in the wall of the building. St. Louis could see a soft light, a lamp lit in the rear of the room beyond the doors. He looked around, trying to get his bearings, and then he realized that this courtyard must be attached to the baby house, that this must be Hoffman's private courtyard, giving out from his rooms.

He tensed when he heard the sound of a door opening and, a moment later, closing in the room inside the French doors. He heard Hoffman's voice. He could not make out what he said, though it had the intonation of a greeting to someone familiar. Hoffman's shape—loosening the tie at his throat—crossed before the French doors and then crossed back again and moved deeper into the room, or perhaps into another room. It was hard to tell.

He looked up. Capuchin had not moved.

He did not want to be caught up in this tree. Hoffman obviously had someone there with him. He reached up a hand and spoke quietly to the monkey, but at the approach of St. Louis's fingers through the leaves, the monkey screamed—a terrible ululation, female-sounding.

St. Louis snatched back his hand in anger. *That* would give them away. Well, the monkey was none of his responsibility. He shifted his weight on the branch—one leg had gone to sleep beneath him—and began to try to back out of the tree.

And then she was there beneath him, standing in the courtyard a step or two beyond the open French doors. She wore her old silk robe, and her hair was untied, as if she were relaxed, at home. He could see that her feet were bare.

"What was *that*?" He saw Hoffman come up behind her, put his hands on her shoulders, and look out into the courtyard with her. "What on *earth* was that?"

Caro didn't say anything. St. Louis felt as if the air between them were evaporating in sheets; with every moment he was being revealed more clearly to her.

"Well, I'd say it was a monkey," Caro said quietly at last.

"A monkey!"

"You sound surprised."

"Well, shouldn't I be?"

"It *is* a fair," she said, reminding him. St. Louis heard the tone of her voice—she was teasing now, sweet and familiar. And yet suddenly he knew she had seen him. He closed his eyes.

"Haven't you heard the lions roar, either?" he heard her ask Hoffman.

"No, I have not." St. Louis opened his eyes to see Hoffman turning Caro toward him, running his hands down her body. "Do they sound as dreadful as this thing you claim is a monkey?"

"Oh, it *is* a monkey," Caro said. "I'm familiar with them."

St. Louis saw her begin to push Hoffman gently back inside.

"I'd know that monkey anywhere," she said, more loudly. "He will go home soon, I think, back where he belongs."

And then he could not hear them anymore, for the door had shut and the figures of Caro and Hoffman had passed beyond his sight.

He sat there for a moment on the branch. He looked at his hands in the darkness; black hair grew over them toward the knuckles. He thought of the hair in his ears and nose, thought of the thick hair on his back and how it spread scantily over his rear end, thought of his short, ugly body, the too-long arms, the Neanderthal brow. One day earlier in the summer he had wandered into the Man Measuring Lab, an exhibit sponsored by researchers at Harvard. Fairgoers volunteered to step up and be examined—the size and formation of their skulls, the width of their noses, the texture of their skin. All this information the scientists jotted down; at the end of the summer they would produce a picture of the era's average new man and woman, corrected by the information of the present. On an im-

pulse, St. Louis had stepped up to be counted. He'd half expected to be turned away, but the serious-faced young man had
seated him in a chair, wound the pleasantly cool tape round
his head, stepped away to make a mark in a notebook.

St. Louis watched the young man's face. He was a handsome
boy, well kept, with short wavy hair the color of fresh butter
combed back neatly. He was probably brilliant, a wonderful
career ahead of him.

"So, tell me," St. Louis asked abruptly. "Just how far off the
curve am I?"

The young man had not looked up from his notebook. "We
don't release that kind of information, sir."

"Why not?" St. Louis had felt outrage—not at this boy,
with his manner too distant for his age, but at himself, as if his
body's failure to grow were a betrayal, a public humiliation. He
had not even been worth getting to full size. *Just tell me,* he
wanted to say. *Am I a freak?*

No, not a freak, he thought now. *An animal. A monkey to be
sent home.*

And he had to squeeze his eyes shut against the pain of
what she had said. For there had been no fondness in her tone.

Though why would there be? She thought he had been spy-
ing on her.

But that was wrong.

He, too, could be angry now, he thought, scraping his hand
painfully against the trunk of the tree as he came down. He
began to hurry down the alley and away.

But before he'd even had time to think of what he had seen,
let alone how he would answer to Caro, he found himself on his
hands and knees; he had tripped over something soft and
weighty at his feet.

And when he turned the man over and put his ear to his

chest, the old organ-grinder's face flashed up at him, empty as a pool of water.

And then the man's face awoke suddenly, and St. Louis drew a breath.

The man shifted, groaned, tried to raise himself on one elbow, and fell back again.

St. Louis put out restraining hands. "Don't move, old father," he said. "Don't worry. It's all right."

Up in the tree overhead, he heard the monkey's scrambling descent.

He looked up from where he knelt, saw the monkey's white face, worried, peering down through the leaves. The organ-grinder muttered something unintelligible, grimaced under his thick mustache. St. Louis saw a trickle of blood move from a dark wound on the old man's head down his temple as he shifted. He smelled foully of liquor.

St. Louis stood up, breathing hard; he waited only an instant, and then he crossed the alley to Hoffman's gate and knocked loudly at the planked door.

He had not planned to run before the door could be opened, but his feet took him away, fast. When he gained the corner, though, he stopped and hesitated. He looked back in time to see the door swing open, light falling into the alley. He saw Hoffman step forward into the light and then saw him stop as he discovered the body of the organ-grinder and then come to his knees at the old man's side. As Hoffman looked up again, St. Louis pressed back around the corner.

He leaned back against the stone wall and closed his eyes. He could almost hear Hoffman thinking, *How comes this man to be lying here in the alley behind my garden in the night? Who knocked on my door and summoned me? Who knew I was here?*

But Caro would know the answers to those questions.

It was almost two hours before the old organ-grinder could be treated—Dr. Hoffman cleaned his head wound with antiseptic, stitched him up neatly—and carried away by the ambulance to the hospital. Kneeling at the man's side, Dr. Hoffman had ascertained that he was mostly drunk; he had fallen in the alley, obviously, occasioning the blow to his head. But he was old and in poor health—confused and upset and breathing shallowly. Dr. Hoffman judged him a good candidate for a heart attack and considered him lucky. Whoever had roused Dr. Hoffman had probably saved the man's life.

"I wonder—" he said to Caro when he returned to his rooms after seeing the ambulance off. "It's strange, don't you think? Did someone know I was here? Who would have knocked at the gate and then run off like that?"

Caro said nothing but came over and sat by him on the bed. She had gotten dressed while he was gone.

Hoffman looked over at her and then reached and took her hands. Why was she dressed now? Was she planning on leaving? What an upsetting night it had been; he was used to practicing medicine in the confines of his own nursery. Yet this summer he seemed to have done a lot of kneeling in the street. He kneaded her hands with his thumbs, almost absently, and then leaned over and put his arms around her. "Don't go," he said. "Don't go because of this."

"You should sleep."

He breathed in the fragrance of her hair. "I'm wide awake now." He sat back and released her shoulders, but he kept her hands in his own. She stood up after a minute, gently pulling her hands from his, and walked toward the doors that led out into the courtyard.

He watched her. "What is it?"

"The monkey's still up there, in the tree," she said.

She would leave, he thought. She would leave him now, just when he most wanted the comfort of her body beside him, the astonishing balm of her presence—pure beauty applied to whatever was difficult or ugly, canceling it out like an eclipse. Tonight's business with that sad old man—it had upset her. Suddenly, he felt the weight of all that was around them: the fair with its tragic, doomed population of itinerants and freaks, its tricks of light and games of chance, its furious, breakneck demonstration of scientific witness and victory. *See? See what we have accomplished? See how the world and all its invisible forces comes under our dominion?* Yet all of it—everyone at the fair that summer, his own tiny babies and even the fair's immortal heroes, like General Italo Balbo, who landed his roaring Italian air armada in the churning waters of the Century of Progress, completing the greatest mass flight in the history of aviation—all of it felt to him vulnerable and fragile. Beyond the familiar horizon, which they could understand and measure, lay an unknown place, a forbidden place, he thought, so full of mystery and light and dark that all the brilliance of the Century of Progress would seem in comparison like the faraway, weakening light of dead stars, nothing but a memory, and then nothing but a story someone had told again and again but one day found they had forgotten altogether.

How much time did they have left?

The summer was dwindling to only a few short weeks; soon he would have to start making preparations with Dr. Ludwig for the infants who had no homes. They had talked about it briefly tonight, in fact. Soon he would have to make preparations for . . . for the future. He felt bewildered for a moment. Where would they go? he wondered, thinking of himself and Caro. What would she do?

Suddenly he stood up. "Caro."

She turned and faced him.

"I have something to show you," he said, and held out his hand.

He did not introduce her immediately to the nurses on shift, nor to Dr. Ludwig's young resident, but led her instead to the center of the room, his hand under her arm. A nurse, a clipboard in her hand, began to approach them, an expression of surprise on her face, but he stopped her with a look—*Just a minute*—and she turned around, her head bowed deferentially. He wanted Caro to have a chance to look about her undisturbed for a minute.

Here was his place.

It was strange to try to see the nursery as she must be seeing it, for the first time—the rows of boxy incubators lining the walls, the white rocking chairs scattered here and there over the gleaming tile floor, the glass-shaded lamps turned low. In the incubators, the babies slept, barely visible except as tiny white loaves. It was very quiet. The silence he'd always associated with the vigilance required of him and his staff was complete; even the nurses, stunned into speechlessness by his arrival in the middle of the night with Caro at his side (did they know who she was? Did anyone recognize her in her man's trousers and loose white shirt?) made no sound as they moved quietly from incubator to incubator. He glanced at Caro; her expression was wary, unsure, and he began, in the face of her doubt, to hear the silence as she must be hearing it. Could she pick out, as he could, the mechanical breathing of the incubators, the quiet noise of a page being turned across the room, an instrument striking a single note against the edge of a metal tray, the gurgle of water? And what else? And then he realized that there was nothing else, and he stood in the center of his nursery as if he were a stranger. The silence here was profound, almost dreadful—the silence at the brink of a cliff. Nowhere in this room were the small comforting noises of the world, the world he suddenly remembered falling asleep in so ardently as a child, his high-ceilinged room in Paris, with the sound of horses' hooves receding on the cobbles outside, the distant notes of the piano from his mother's sitting room downstairs, the front door opening and closing to the street, pigeons rustling in the ivy. How clear it all was. Where had it gone?

He looked around him, appalled at the stark poverty of what he had created—the incubators gleamed like ovens, he saw, shocked. The babies slept on behind the dark glass doors, and slept on, and slept on.

If only one of them would wake. Then he could show her the world.

He led her across the room to the hatbox baby's incubator. They stood before the glass doors together—he could feel the heat of her arm under his fingers—and it seemed to him that they stood there like two pilgrims, two children themselves, unsure of what they would see. Where was the comfort he'd felt in this particular child's presence, the sense that his efforts had not gone unappreciated, and yet that they were not the deciding factor, that something else was controlling this baby's fate.

He put his hand on Caro's back.

"An orphan," he whispered to her.

And then the child moved; a tiny hand flashed loose from its wrappings.

He heard the sharp intake of Caro's breath.

Dr. Hoffman smiled. The child had greeted them, he thought. It had heard his voice. And though the notion was foolish and sentimental, it pleased him to entertain it and be moved by it. He let go of Caro, stepped forward, and opened the doors; a whiff of oxygen met his nostrils. He lifted the baby in his arms and was reassured by so much that was suddenly familiar and right—the weight of the baby, the silky smoothness of its cheek, the smell of its skin. He turned around to show the baby to Caro, to put it in her arms, for it had folded itself up deliciously (that was the word, *delicious!* What a surprise, to discover this!) into his embrace.

But Caro had stepped backward and was looking away from him, her hands in her pockets.

He smiled at her, but she did not return his look. He waited a moment, puzzled. He glanced at the nurses; he could tell they were purposely avoiding looking in his and Caro's direction. He could not insist, though, with them in the room.

"Caro," he said softly.

She looked toward him once and then glanced away. "Leo," she said, "I'm sorry. It isn't what I expected. Or it is—I can't tell."

He held the baby. "What do you mean?"

She said nothing.

"Come on," he said. "He's my favorite. Come and hold him."

She turned toward him with a look of pleading; her expression was anguished. He felt the smile leave his face.

"Another time," she said. "Please."

He turned around and put the baby back. Caro was close to tears, and he felt mortified, hurrying her out of the room. What would they say behind his back now? He could not even stop and speak to the resident.

They reached his rooms. Caro went ahead of him and stepped out into the garden.

He waited in the doorway. He did not understand what had happened.

Finally she turned around, showing him a beautiful smile through her tears. "You won't understand," she said. "I don't understand. It's just—I'm forty-five years old, Leo. I won't ever have—" She stopped and made a helpless gesture. "What a life I've led."

He stepped down into the courtyard and put his arms around her.

"I thought I wanted to see it: Where you work. What you do. The babies," she said into his shirt, more quietly now. "But it frightened me."

My God. You're wrong, he thought. *You could have this so easily.* And yet he knew that wasn't true. It wouldn't be *easy.*

But he would have asked her then; it was almost on his lips to say it.

"It's so late." She stepped back, away from him. "I need to sleep."

Silence hung between them.

She walked to the gate and opened it.

"Caro . . ." What was she saying to him? Was she saying good-bye? Was she saying no?

"Leo. Sleep well," she said. And then she was gone.

He stood in the empty courtyard.

It was so much more complicated than he could ever have imagined; for he could never have imagined loving her to begin with. He had been right that what she did, how she led her life, was an obstacle between them, not only for him, who could not bear to think of how she disrobed, how she danced for other men—all the *years* of it—but for her, too. And yet it was also the explanation of her attraction—the surprise of her, to find this woman he now loved behind the common seduction of her beauty.

Common or uncommon? No, now he knew. It was uncommon. There was no one else like her.

How would this ever be mended? And which of them, he thought, pulling out a chair and sitting down, which of them had the most to lose?

He took off his glasses and put his head in his hands. He could not even begin to reckon the cost of her loss to him, for he was used to dealing with things that were small—tiny babies, four-inch vials of milk, beds no longer than a foot, tiny shoes that rode on the ball of your thumb.

This, the grief he felt now, was beyond his experience, he thought. He had no words at all for something this large.

THIRTEEN

For a few weeks, it was perfect. St. Louis brought steaming trays of hot cocoa and cinnamon rolls from the Café de la Paix for the nurses and Alice in the mornings and stayed to watch the babies being bathed and fed, sometimes helping Alice, who talked to him while she worked, explaining to him what she did, how she moved the babies' arms and legs, tested their strength and resistance, exercised their tiny bodies. He loved it all—the clear, warm water full of sunlight from the high transom windows, the babies' cries, their shining skin. The infants no longer looked sickly to him; they seemed heroic.

After the last afternoon showings he came back and rocked; in a week he had held all the babies, though he moved instinctively, always, to the hatbox baby, once Louise had pointed him out, and loved him especially, his dark blue eyes, his mobile little face. He took him in his arms every chance he got, reveling in the smell and weight and feel of him. On Hoffman's orders, several infants who had grown large and vigorous enough had been deemed sufficiently strong to move out of the incubators and now slept in rolling bassinets. The hatbox baby, he saw one day when Nan Silverman weighed him, was over five pounds, gaining on six, and looked almost like a proper baby, as he thought of it, in its new open bed. Alice called him a record-breaker.

He left the nursery while the public showings were going on but sometimes returned to stay through dinner and the evening hours, running back to the Lido at midnight for Caro's last show, to shoo away the men who lingered at the stage door, waiting for her to come out and give autographs or, they hoped, other favors. Over lunch at the café every Friday, he sharpened his pencil and did the books for Caro. She had made more money this summer than any before.

His conversation with Caro, the day after the incident in the tree, had gone smoothly enough. He had made his explanations, and she had accepted them quietly with what he thought was a surprising lack of resistance or spirit. There had been no fight between them, though he had expected one, still wounded by her remark about the monkey. He had not reminded her of it, though; she could probably recall it well enough herself, and he supposed she was sorry for it, though she didn't say so. Instead he had asked—given her friendship with Hoffman, he explained—if she would say something to the doctor about St. Louis's interest in the babies. "Put in a good word, you know," he'd asked shyly, sitting across from her on the hassock in her dressing room that afternoon. She had said she would, and apparently Hoffman had been told, for the doctor greeted him cordially, although formally, when he saw him, though he seemed inclined to avoid conversation with him.

"It's funny how things work out, isn't it?" he'd said to Caro. "You and the baby doctor."

Caro had looked up at him from her dressing table. She looked tired to him. "Funny?" she said. "I guess so."

But Caro herself, St. Louis could not figure out. They rarely saw each other now; he was so busy at the baby house. And she offered him nothing in the way of information or confidence. Once, though, he had made himself ask her about Hoffman. It seemed too important a topic for them never to have discussed it.

"What's going to happen when it's over?" he'd said. They had been sitting on the pier one Sunday afternoon, looking out over the lake—a rare outing for the two of them. Caro had stopped performing on Sundays; the fair board had been outraged and threatened breach of contract, but when she said she would pull out altogether, contract or no contract, they relented. No matter how much money she might have to turn over if they won a suit against her, it could never be as much as she would earn by staying. And there was next summer to think of, too, when the fair would have its second and last season. The board did not want to risk losing her engagement for next summer.

"Do you want to go back to New York with him?" he asked her. He'd passed on booking requests to her, but she had made no decisions, as far as he knew. Before, she'd always had plans.

"He hasn't asked me."

St. Louis stole a look at her profile. This was new, Caro waiting to be asked. She stared off toward the horizon.

"Oh." He found himself fumbling for words. "But do you *want* to?"

She didn't answer him. "What's happened to you?" she said instead. "Remember that day you told me you didn't know what was wrong? But something's changed. You're better. Happy."

"I know." St. Louis watched a distant sailboat steering toward them, the clean triangle of its white sail and red hull making it seem like a child's toy boat. "I think it's the babies." He remembered with some embarrassment what he'd said about wanting to be a doctor. "I just feel useful, is all."

Caro did not reply to this right away. For a few minutes they watched the water together, the glistening expanse. Nearby, a man leaned over the railing of the pier, holding on to the legs of a sturdy little redheaded boy who chortled with pleasure.

"And what will *you* do when it's over?" she said.

St. Louis looked at her again. Her question—it implied that they would not be together. He was shocked, for though he had thought it himself, he had never expected to be dismissed from her company. And yet it sounded as if she was assuming it anyway.

"The fair," she repeated. "When it's over, what will you do?"

"Are you telling me I am free to choose?" He did not want to sound angry—after all, he had been contemplating such a change himself all summer—and yet he heard the edge in his voice. Why did sadness so often disguise itself as anger? he wondered.

"You have always been free to choose," she said.

It was true, he thought, that he had come to the end of his role as Caro's protector. *They* had come to the end of it together, perhaps. Sully did the job just as well, and he'd follow Caro anywhere. They could easily hire a bookkeeper to watch the money. Yet it was also true that he had nowhere to go. This came as a surprise to him. He supposed he could follow Hoffman back to Coney Island and do there what he was doing here—rocking the babies, enjoying Alice's company, Louise's—and yet it was not exactly the right solution. He would be as adrift there as he was here, and that was the problem. Being adrift. Before, Caro had always kept him from feeling that way. Now he believed she was suggesting that the arrangement between them—the unspoken bond that kept them together—had already mysteriously dissolved. From now on, if they were to stay together, they would have to choose each other.

He blinked at the water, which was suddenly blinding to him, light assailing them like fat from a fire. He put up his arm. It was too bright here. He could not see clearly.

"There's only two weeks left," Caro said, and suddenly he hated the reasonable tone in her voice.

"I know that," he said. "You don't have to tell me that."

She shrugged, put a hand on his shoulder to help her climb to her feet. He looked up to her as she stood beside him, waiting. She seemed to tower over him; her dark hair, full of a spectrum of light, fell partway over her face.

"Well, we have a little time left," she said, and reached a hand down toward him.

He took it and held on for a minute before allowing her to help pull him up. He remembered holding her hand as a child. He remembered—could he really see this far back?—Caro holding out her arms to him over the pool of the bubbling, steaming spring back on the farm in Pharaoh. "Jump," she had said to him, and he had looked down into the magic water. Would it swallow him? Drown him? Turn him to gold? "Jump, St. Louis!"

And he had jumped then, into her arms.

But it wouldn't be the same now. This time, there were no arms held out to catch him.

It was the hottest day of the summer, August 31, and the headlines were full of tragedy. A Negro child had been hit by a train outside Chicago and killed, his body severed in two. The Yellow River in Shanghai had flooded across endless green plains of rice and countless villages of Chinese peasants; thousands had died.

The new Federal Home Owner's Loan Corporation had opened in Chicago, and seventeen thousand desperate people had shown up to apply for assistance on the first day; there had been riots in the street.

Nazi storm troopers passing in review in Berlin had heard another sermon attacking Jews.

A Bible salesman had killed the owner of a small hotel by beating him over the head with a club and then slicing his skin to ribbons.

A child had died of tetanus after being hit on the head by his mother's slipper, thrown from across the room to stop the child from crying.

Cotton growers were burning bales to raise prices.

Twin sisters, examined by alienists after they had shot their own mother, had been judged by the insanity commission and sent to an asylum.

A review of high school bands at the fair had turned into a disaster. One hundred and eighteen children had collapsed under their instruments from the heat, even though it was early in the day; two ambulances had collided on the sizzled, brown grass of the field, trying to get to the victims.

St. Louis had been at the baby house in the morning, but everyone had been in bad spirits. The air-cooling system had broken down, and Hoffman, enraged, had finally gone off to find workmen himself, after his appeals to the maintenance crews had gone unanswered. Apparently, systems all over the fair were breaking down. Hoffman had ordered the transom windows opened and had seen that the wet nurses brought pails of ice into the nursery, where they set up fans to blow over the ice and offer a meager relief. He had been worried about the heat for the babies and had blown up at Alice before leaving to go seek help.

"It will be on *their* heads, *their* heads," he had fumed, shrugging off his gown and searching around irritably for his jacket.

St. Louis had noticed that Hoffman never went anywhere unless he was impeccably attired.

"We can keep them cool enough," Alice had said, trying to be reasonable, though her own uniform was wet with sweat in the back. She looked uglier than usual, St. Louis had thought with pity. A red face only heightened the crude quality of her features; she looked like a giantess. "We'll increase their baths."

"You have not got enough ice," Hoffman had said. "You will run out." And then he had left.

St. Louis had done what he could. He paid the waiters at the Café de la Paix to trundle over cakes of ice on dollies, but it was so hot that they dripped all over the floors before the waiters could get them into tubs, upsetting Alice. He had bathed several infants himself; Alice and Nan were too busy with the fans, with the increased number of baths prescribed by Hoffman, and with two complaining wet nurses, who claimed their milk had dried up because it was so hot. Even the babies were upset, irritable and restless. Nan and the other nurses finally persuaded Alice to close the nursery to the public. Alice, who did not like taking such a step without Hoffman, had worried and worried over it until even St. Louis was annoyed with her. But when Hoffman had not returned by eleven that morning, she sent Louise outside to go put up a sign on the door.

Louise was gone for several minutes. Alice, who had been weighing the nursery's second set of twins, and girl and a boy with disconcertingly full heads of shiny black hair, had finally dumped them unceremoniously into St. Louis's lap and was going out to see what was keeping her so long when Louise came back into the nursery.

There was a young woman with her, standing uncertainly behind her.

Louise waited at the door. The young woman—blond and pretty and neatly dressed, though not expensively, St. Louis thought—waited behind Louise, looking around with anxious, hopeful eyes.

"Alice!" Louise called across the room, her voice too loud and peremptory, and crooked a finger in Alice's direction, summoning her. Everyone stopped and turned. "Would you come over here a minute?"

And as Alice walked across the room, St. Louis found himself suddenly holding the babies so tightly that one of them began to cry.

The young woman's voice was low as she spoke to Alice, giving a long explanation during which the young woman broke down several times. Louise, whom Alice had failed to send away for some reason—perhaps out of her own surprise at what was unfolding— stood by, patting the girl's shoulder possessively. St. Louis saw Alice nod her head several times and bring her hand slowly to her forehead to wipe away the sweat. The young woman kept her eyes on Alice's face as the two spoke; St. Louis watched her, slowing his rocking until he had come to a complete stop, leaning forward in his chair, straining to hear.

And then he saw them both turn and saw Alice point to the hatbox baby—his baby, *his beautiful hatbox baby*—and saw the young woman's hand fly to her mouth. Louise scuttled away to fetch a tissue, returned, offered a chair, a glass of water. The young woman sat, holding up her hand, asking for time, staring in the direction of the bassinet in which the hatbox baby slept. Alice stood by, a sentinel, refusing judgment, wiping her own face.

She had seen this before, St. Louis thought. She had seen babies reclaimed at the last minute, before it was too late.

His hatbox baby. His hatbox baby would go.

And then Alice glanced back and met St. Louis's eyes.

What passed between them, St. Louis thought later, was a kind of apology, each of them apologizing for being unable to prevent what would happen next.

"Why won't you?" St. Louis tried to control his voice, but it came out raw and furious, anyway. "Why? Give me one good reason."

They were up in the Ferris wheel, in the middle of the night. St. Louis had said he needed to talk to her alone, and Caro had proposed the Ferris wheel. "Maybe there'll be some air up there," she'd said wearily. "Come on, Sully. Take us up."

"I've never asked you for *anything*!" He knew he shouldn't yell at her, but he couldn't help it. She sat there as if he'd asked her something completely unimportant, like whether she'd lend him a five. He wanted to hit her.

"You have to give me a reason," he said, trying to keep his voice calm. "I said I'd take care of it. You don't have to do anything, if you don't want. *I* know how to look after a baby. Caro, please. No one would let me adopt one, but Hoffman would just *give* you one. You know he would! There's five or six headed for the orphanage. No one wants them. But I do. *I do.*"

Caro still said nothing. St. Louis stared at her for a moment and then looked away down at the fairgrounds. He thought of the sight-seeing plane, a big-bellied Sikorsky amphibian, that had crashed a few days before in Glenview, after a failed landing on the lake. He thought about the plane's wings mowing down the buildings below, slicing through the tilting surfaces and soft materials of the walls, hacking them to bits. It was all made out of nothing anyway, he thought. Nothing but light and air.

"Caro," he said, turning back to her. "Answer me."

"We're not the sort of people to raise children." She didn't look at him.

"What do you mean?" He stood up, holding on to the bar in front of him.

"Sit down." Caro reached up and pulled him back into his seat.

He shrugged away from her. "Tell me what you mean. What's the right sort of person? You're not the right sort of person? I'm not? Why not? We're a lot better than plenty of people out there who—who starve their children or beat them or send them off to work in factories." He'd heard Roosevelt talk about this in his radio addresses; St. Louis and Caro had always agreed with Roosevelt about child labor. "We wouldn't ever do that! We'd just—we'd just *love* a baby, Caro," he finished help-lessly. "We'd only *love* a baby."

She said nothing, and in her silence he felt the possibility of cruelty forming itself into words in his mouth. "Is it because you take your clothes off and dance around before a bunch of slobbering men?" he said then, staring at her. "Is it because you're a *stripper*? Or because I'm a freak?" he said. "Which is it? Which is worse?"

Caro did not look at him. She seemed not to have registered the insult of his words; or perhaps she had said them already to herself, he thought.

"Babies should have families, real families." Caro's eyes seemed to be fixed on the fairgrounds below, the chaotic grid of light beneath them. "Babies should have mothers who stay home and wear aprons and cook supper and wash diapers and bake apple pies. And fathers who go off to work and come home and cut the grass and listen to the radio. That's not us, St. Louis. It's not, and it never will be."

St. Louis clenched the railing of the seat in front of him. *I thought we* were *a family,* he wanted to say. *We* are *a family.*

But he said nothing else.

He leaned out the window instead and called down to the ground, his voice bitter. "Sully! Sully!" He saw Sully move into the light and look up at them. "Cut this thing off," St. Louis called down. "We're finished."

As the car jerked forward and began its slow, swinging descent, he looked over the lights of the Century of Progress. *How small and foolish it all is,* he thought at first, *like a bunch of building blocks knocked over by a child's foot.* But as they drew closer to the ground, he was struck once again, almost despite himself, by the magic of the lights. It was so easy, after all, to allow yourself to be seduced by it, the innocent, hopeful play of color over the streets and up the walls of the monuments, the caressing charm of the lights' weightless touch, how they stole into the car in which he and Caro rode now, sliding a rainbow of color over their faces. He looked down at his hands, saw them transformed to red and then blue and then green and then a blinding yellow like the sun itself, as if anyone could be changed in just a moment. Why had he resisted it for so long? he wondered. What's the harm in it?

But then he told himself what he needed to hear in order to steady himself and fix his purpose.

It's only sleight of hand, he said to himself. *It's nothing but a trick. Now you see it, now you don't.*

Well, watch this, he thought. *Watch this.*

Pharaoh, Virginia

September 1933

FOURTEEN

The first night back in Pharaoh, St. Louis walked out beyond the lights of the farmhouse and lay down in the darkness of the meadow, the hatbox baby asleep on his chest. The hollow spines of late-summer hay, still uncut though it was September now, cracked beneath him as he settled himself on the ground, the baby held against his chest with one arm. When he closed his eyes, his head at rest at last on a pillow of matted grass, and cupped his hands around the funny knobs of the infant's heels, he took comfort in the rustling, whispering barricade that concealed them.

The meadow smelled so familiar that he was surprised; when so much else had changed, how could it be that this scent—sweet and faintly peppery—should have stayed the same all these years? And it was absurd to feel safe here just because he was lying in the grass, hidden from view; he understood that. Why, anyone could walk up to the worn porch steps of the farmhouse now and rouse his furious, incoherent uncle; Warren might be loose in the head, but when St. Louis had come up the hill to the farmhouse earlier that day, the baby in his arms, there'd been no question about Warren's ability to see what was before him—though he'd been wrong about one thing.

"That's Caroline's bastard baby," Warren Day had shouted at St. Louis from behind the screen door. "You don't fool me, St. Louis. That's my daughter's bastard baby."

Warren himself wasn't likely to answer a knock on his door in any case. It would be Louise who would come to stand at the bottom of the stairs, her wrapper tied loosely around her waist, her hands on her hips.

That last day in Chicago, when he had pulled her outside the baby house and shown her the wad of bills, she'd promised to help him, but only for a little while. "Hey," she'd added, seeing his face. "You never know. Maybe they won't even guess where you are. Maybe they won't care."

But of course they would care, St. Louis thought. Hoffman especially would care very much. And it wouldn't take Caro a minute to guess where he'd gone. That's how stupid he was.

He pictured Hoffman at the farmhouse door, rigid and enraged and—worst of all—disgusted, turning to follow Louise's finger, pointing down out of the pale, waxy light of the kitchen into the dark, rustling meadow below the house.

There they are. The snake who stole into your nursery and the baby he took with him when he left.

All the same, despite what he knew to be true, St. Louis did feel safe. The grass swayed around him in the darkness, making a dry noise, a low, steady breathing. He heard the wind, coming from a long way away over the mountains, arrive at the meadow's edge and begin to move toward him, bowing the tips of the grasses, which brushed against one another with the delicate sound of paper rustling. He cupped a hand over the baby's soft, warm head, the head that fit so perfectly in his palm. The child stirred gently but slept on over his heart, a small, significant weight.

St. Louis tilted his head back and gazed up into the sky. Motionless bunches of yellow night clouds hung there in the darkness, stars shining far away in the black depths. What a place the sky would be with no stars. Earlier this summer, he'd been to an Indian wedding at the fair; an old man there had told him a pretty story about the stars. The nuptials of Long Grass and Dipper of Water—St. Louis had no idea if those were their real names or whether they had others: Sam, perhaps, or Sid? Irene? Mary?—had been grand and ceremonial, staged to attract crowds to the Seminole encampment, where tourists might buy a pair of pretty beaded moccasins for a girl, or a tiny painted drum of stiff white birch bark for a boy. But late that evening, after the wedding, after the fairgoers had all gone home, the Indians had held their own party—the wedding had been not just a gimmick for the crowds, but a real love match, too. A circle of picnic tables had been set up on the brown grass beyond the bright circle of tepees; trays of roasted corn and bottles of liquor were set out on newspaper, starlight overhead. Around midnight, over a tablecloth damp with spilled beer and littered with overturned bottles and the grinning, half-moon rinds of cherry-colored melons, an old Indian man had sat down beside him. While they looked up into the night sky over Lake Michigan together, the old man had told him a story about how Indians turned into stars when they died, generations reuniting in the folds of the constellations' robes.

St. Louis watched the stars now from where he lay hidden in the meadow. The smells around him were growing faintly sour. He remembered this change from his childhood; as the heat of the day evaporated, it took with it the last residual sweetness, replacing it with something cold and stony. He sniffed, rubbed a hand over the baby's back. Being a star—now that was a cold, beautiful fate, he thought, his gaze slowly traversing the sky overhead. But wouldn't he make for a clumsy-looking star? Short and thick and as ugly in the hereafter as now, holding on to the yellow night clouds like a man trying not to fall overboard?

He patted the baby's back. The child gave a sigh, contracted itself against his chest, nestling in. Overhead, stars appeared and disappeared.

According to the old Indian's story, one day, if he could keep this baby, he'd have a pretty bit of light for company in the souls' endless watch over the fate of the world.

Why, give him ten babies, and he'd be a galaxy!

That was a thought. He looked up, blinking; children in twinkling white shifts ran in and out of the barn's dark door, ran up the hill toward him with flowers in their hands, with the discovered eggs of the sneaky guinea hen, with white pebbles in their palms. He stepped down from the porch, stooped to open his arms and take them in, so many of them, all his beautiful children running toward him.

But the world worked by a strange justice. They wouldn't let him keep this baby, much less let him raise ten children, even though nobody wanted the incubator babies; people thought they'd be ruined for having come so early. They seemed strange to the men and women who paid money to come see them in Hoffman's beautiful incubators—little half-formed things, unable to live in the air of the real world. He'd thought they were strange once, too.

But now, one baby, ten babies . . . he'd overheard Alice and Nan talking; there were at least six who had no parents willing

to claim them, even with so many people gawking and marveling
—little Pearl, sweet Henry, tiny, blind Bernice, poor ruined
Robert.

Why hadn't he taken one of those? They might have let him
keep one of those.

But he'd wanted the hatbox baby.

He was responsible for the hatbox baby. He'd saved the
baby's life once, in a way—steering him into Hoffman's hands.
And now, shouldn't that life be his to protect and cherish
forever?

Shouldn't it?

An owl's call floated down through the darkness over the
meadow from the far-off stand of honey locusts and hickories
at the foot of High Peak, black against the mountain's gray rise.

Oh, they'd take the baby away, for certain.

He closed his eyes. The baby's back rose and fell lightly
under his hand, steady as a heartbeat. A whirring began, low
in the grass near his feet, and then stopped as if silenced by a
hand.

What had made him think he could get away with this?

He had left Chicago three days before, boarding the
night train in a frenzy of fear and haste with Louise and the
two babies, her baby and the stolen baby, one a fat, greasy-
looking child with small pig eyes, and his, his own hatbox
baby, with the perfect tiny hands and ears and toes. It had
been so easy to walk out with the baby, just waiting until the
nurses' backs were turned, substituting a rolled blanket under
the coverings in the baby's bed, just to give them time enough
to get away. Louise had complained that she hadn't been able
to pack properly—someone would have noticed—but he'd as-
sured her that he'd buy her whatever she wanted.

Twice, waiting for the train to leave the station, he thought he'd heard Caro's voice. And once he thought he'd seen Hoffman, the doctor's calm shattered by the duplicity of the crime against him, running down the platform after them; but it had only been a man with a satchel.

The train had lingered at the station for an interminable time.

Go, go, *go*! St. Louis had willed it to move, staring hatefully through the dirty compartment window at the slow-moving porters with their white teeth and black, gleaming faces, milling purposelessly on the platform, lit with trembling saucers of white light.

But when their car lurched forward at last, he had not been ready. He had stumbled and caught at the rack over their heads with his free hand. The baby, held against his chest with one arm, had begun to mewl.

"Give him here," Louise had said, the first of her unexpected kindnesses. He hadn't even had to ask.

She'd sat up and laid her own infant in the basket at her feet. Under a light blanket, she put the hatbox baby to her breast instead, twitched at a corner of it to conceal herself, and then leaned back, yawning. She wore a black straw hat with a queer false set of dark bangs attached to the brim, and a cream-colored ribbon around the crown. When she nestled back against the seat, the hat tipped forward over her eyes in a clownish way. Louise wasn't pretty, St. Louis had thought, looking at her; her skin was thickly freckled, and she had wiry, dark hair the dull color of walnuts, and rolls of mottled pink flesh at her neck. But she was a sport. Five hundred dollars had bought him a sport, at least for a while.

The first night on the train, because he wanted to show Louise his largesse, wanted to show her that he could look after her, even if it was only a business arrangement they had, they'd eaten chop

suey from waxy paper boxes on their laps, thirty-five cents a carton. He'd bought them each a glass of buttermilk at ten cents
apiece, and fifteen-cent slices of yellow layer cake. He'd saved
her half his buttermilk and his whole slice of cake. "Because
you're feeding them, too," he'd said, leaning over the babies,
which were asleep between them, and offering her his glass.

She'd shrugged but had taken the glass. She smiled at him
after finishing the buttermilk. "I don't know where you got
them, because you don't look the type, no offense," she said,
"but you have nice manners for—"

He stood up too fast, spilling his supper carton.

She looked up at him, a stain the color of liver spreading up
her neck. "I didn't mean—"

"It's all right," he said.

He'd gone for a walk down the swinging body of the train,
standing deafened for several minutes in the dark between clat-
tering cars. The force of the cool night air hitting his face made
his eyes water. *What do you know?* he asked himself furiously.
What do you know? Nothing. Over and over again he felt the
weight of the money crushed into his pocket. When his fingers
encountered the bills, they were soft as silk, and tempting.

When he returned to their car, Louise was finishing his
cake. "You know what I want now?" she said, bending over
and lifting up the little shirt stretched tight over her baby's fat
stomach to delicately wipe her mouth. The pinprick of light
from the fixture above her swept down her spine and rolled
back again like a marble as she sat up. "I want a Minnehaha
Punch. Or"—her eyes lit up—"a Pedigree Pick-Me-Up! You
have one of those this summer?" She snapped her fingers.
"Lemon, sugar, bourbon, and *an egg,* strained over ice." Her
wet mouth made an egg-shaped hole. "And I'd like baked ham
with champagne sauce."

If he'd put anything more into his stomach, he would have thrown it all up from nerves, so he'd said nothing. At last she'd turned and stared out the window into the wide darkness of the Indiana cornfields rushing past them.

But he was just waiting, waiting to cross the churning water of the Ohio River, waiting for the sound of the train wheels going across the bridge, telling him he was near home.

Louise tried again, one last time that night before they slept. "You ever have the raisin pie at the Hall of Religion?" She turned away from the window to face him; her eyes were bulgy, like guppies' eyes. She stared at him until he'd shaken his head.

"Get it with a Horlicks," she advised him, and he realized she said it as if they were going back someday, as if it would all still be there years from now—the fair and the crowds and the incubator babies—as if nothing they had done, nothing *he* had done, was of any consequence at all.

Lying in the meadow grass now, his first night home with the baby (though was *home* any sort of word to be using under these circumstances? Had it ever been a word he could use?) he lifted one hand from the baby's back and spread his fingers into the darkness above his head. A soft late-summer moon hung above them. Swarms of fireflies gathered briefly at his fingertips, glassy green beads of light that paused and then darted away over the pasture, falling unevenly downhill. The baby stirred under his chin. He tipped his nose and smelled the milk on the baby's head, Louise's milk, and also the scent of the grass around them, stirring invisibly with a faint sound like a dog's sigh, like the breathing sound made by the baby's incubator.

He had stolen a baby.

All the things he had stolen in his life, usually from people who deserved to lose them, or at least could afford to. But never before a baby.

A deer coughed nearby in the woods, down near where the spring used to be, and he tightened his hand over the baby's back, looking up through the film of fireflies that hung above them. His two hands held wide, thumb to thumb, were less than the length of the baby.

The baby stirred under his chin. Was he cold? St. Louis worried about him getting sick, though Louise's rough confidence reassured him. And this morning he thought the baby had actually smiled at him. "Look at that," he'd said to Louise, delighted. "Look. Maybe he'll do it again!"

But Louise had snorted. "Gas," she said expertly. "He's too young to know what he's doing." Then she had softened, seeing St. Louis's face fall. "But you'll be the first, you can be sure of that," she added. "He'll think you're his mother."

St. Louis looked up into the stars and inched the blanket up over the baby's tiny shoulders. He heard the deer cough again, deeper into the woods, looking for water. But the spring was gone now. Dried up, Warren had said.

From the bottom of the hill where the car had stopped to let them off at a little past eleven earlier that day, the grass in the meadow rising to the square white farmhouse had looked to St. Louis like an ocean of gold, the wind parting it into drifts ahead of them. Shifting his case to his other hand and shielding his eyes, he had looked up toward the house, flat as a picture against an almost white sky. He had wanted to feel relief at finally reaching this point; he had been telling himself that he would feel better once they were in Pharaoh. But it had been only a way of helping him maintain his composure along the way, a promised reward at the end of it all. When he did not feel that relief, staring up at his uncle's house at last, he realized that he had always known he wouldn't. That this wasn't the end of anything at all.

But what had he begun?

St. Louis and Louise had stood there for a moment, looking up at the house. And then, as if he had heard the sound of the car's tires grinding away down the gravel road, Warren had darted out onto the porch with a strange, hunched-over motion, as if he were ducking from gunfire.

A new alarm had attached itself to St. Louis along with the rest, clamps fitted to his heart and lungs. They must have wired ahead, Caro and Hoffman. He didn't think Warren had a telephone.

St. Louis has stolen a baby stop. Stop him stop.
Stop him.

In the house on the hill behind him now, Louise and her own gummy-nosed, sweaty baby were asleep. Earlier that evening, she'd handed the hatbox baby to him when she was done feeding him and had buttoned up her dress, folding her large, veined breast casually into a white camisole and stowing it away. She didn't seem embarrassed about St. Louis's seeing her breasts. He supposed that if you made a living as a wet nurse, you got over being modest.

"How long will it be before they come and find you, do you think?" she'd asked him, lying back on the bed, sweat shining on her upper lip.

He'd looked away from her, up to the map of Virginia that was tacked over the bed on the wall behind her. Drooping from a nail in the middle of the map was a piece of red yarn marking the farm's place in Pharaoh, at the base of the Blue Ridge Mountains. The yarn had faded to the color of dried blood.

How much time *did* he have? He knew he should be trying to address this question, to make plans, and he had been trying hard to think about it. But everything he had done seemed so surprising to him, like a crime committed in a dream. He was having trouble focusing on the implications of finally making it to Pharaoh. He was tempted not to answer Louise at all, to put away entirely the struggle of having to think clearly right now.

"Won't *he* mind?" Louise had insisted, gesturing down the shadowy hall to the closed door at the end.

Chips of green paint lay flecking the hall floor where the rain had leaked through once. No one had replastered inside; a stain of concentric gray rings like a tree burl bloomed on the ceiling. Warren had fallen asleep at last earlier that night in a rumple of gray sheets, muttering insults and recriminations, his hands gripped over his head as though he were expecting a blow.

St. Louis had been shocked almost more by the state of his aunt and uncle's bedroom than by the sight of Warren himself, for he remembered his pleasure in the room as it had been when he was a child and his aunt was still alive. She'd kept a rocker by the window and her sewing in a round brown basket on a three-legged table. The blue coverlet had been clean and stretched tight across the bed; the floor was polished with bowling alley wax. On the dresser had stood an amber glass vase his aunt had filled with wildflowers from the pasture. Sometimes, St. Louis and Caro had been allowed to close the canopy of the bed and play at sailing ships there.

Helping Warren into bed that evening, stripping back the sheet and jumping away in disgust as the bugs tumbled out, St. Louis had needed to close his eyes against a sudden dizzying memory of Caro with a knife between her tiny, perfect teeth, coming across the bed toward him on all fours. A pirate.

It was Caro who would come now. St. Louis was sure of that.

This was all her fault, in a way. She could have helped him. She could have, but she wouldn't.

"I know you," Warren had shrilled from behind the screen door when St. Louis and Louise had reached the porch earlier that afternoon.

St. Louis had watched Warren watching them as they'd walked up the long, hot hill from the road, Louise complaining and tripping over the stones in her mules. When they reached the steps, Warren had shaken his finger at them, dancing behind the ripped screen door, screaming in a high, chaotic voice. "You don't fool me, St. Louis. That's her bastard!" And then he had found the breath to pause for emphasis between each word; rage had done it. *"That's Caroline's bastard baby."*

St. Louis had been relieved at first—Warren didn't know *whose* baby it was if he thought it was Caro's—and then appalled. Taking the old man's arm, he'd reeled at Warren's smell of filth and sickness, his thin arm. In the kitchen, Warren had wept. The floor was red with unswept footmarks of Virginia clay. The old man had simply put down his head on the table like a child, obviously relieved that someone had finally come to help him.

Only four years earlier, when St. Louis and Caro had come back briefly for Caro's mother's funeral, Warren had been grim and subdued. But St. Louis would not have predicted this, this complete disintegration, as if Warren had deteriorated from the inside and now the pieces were too changed and diminished to reconnect into even a semblance of who he had once been. Warren didn't make any sense. He talked about people St. Louis didn't know, or about the spring.

"I'll do this floor. You get him upstairs to bed," Louise had said from the kitchen doorway, skepticism and disgust mixed equally in her voice. "He's sick."

Her suitcase had stood on the floor beside her, and she had a baby in each arm.

St. Louis had felt weak. This was where he'd brought them.

But Louise had looked around, practical. "Get me two drawers from a dresser first," she'd ordered, "and clean sheets, if you can find them."

Five hundred dollars had bought him this—she was a sport.

It had been easy enough to come up with the cash. He had taken the money out of his and Caro's private account—there was plenty there—and then, just because he'd felt so heartbroken, he'd liberated the wallets of four drunken gentlemen waiting for a ricksha by the Fountain of Time. Seven hundred dollars later, he had an endless supply of milk from Louise's breasts (until he could find a wet nurse in Pharaoh and Louise could go home to New York) and her willingness to clean up an old man's filth.

St. Louis had stepped carefully across the kitchen over something black and viscous that was pooling under the sink and over the wood floor. He'd had to fight the urge to retch, less at the terrible condition of the house and Warren himself than at the realization of how long it must have been like this to get this bad, and how filthy his own soul felt as a consequence.

Even Caro, blithe as she liked to appear about her father's furious disownment of her and her way of life, would not have wanted this.

"What kind of people are *they,* to let a neighbor get this bad? What's the matter with him *anyway*?" Louise had grumbled, rolling up her sleeves. "Get me a damn bucket. And I'll bet he doesn't have any food, either."

She'd shot St. Louis a look of contempt. These were his people. This is where he came from.

That evening, when Louise lay across the bed in Caro's old room after nursing the baby, St. Louis had looked around, wondering what had become of all Caro's things—the room had been stripped bare. Gone were his and Caro's childish drawings, her butterfly collection and cloth dolls, the wreath of dried flowers that had hung from a peg over her bed.

Louise had found clean sheets in a chest in the hall and had made up the bed. With a length torn from one of the sheets, she had wrapped up the hatbox baby; he looked like a piece of sugar.

"He's all right," she'd said comfortably, handing him over to St. Louis. "Nothing wrong with *this* baby."

A blue drop of milk hung on the baby's cheek. St. Louis wanted to bend down and catch it on his tongue.

Louise had yawned and rolled onto her side, tucked her hands between her knees. St. Louis had looked away from her, gazing up at the map on the wall, his little flag. He'd always meant to mark all the places he went to, but there was only the one pin. Now he couldn't even remember everywhere he'd been, running after Caro.

"Well? Won't he mind us being here? I know what he thinks, even if he *is* crazy," Louise went on sleepily, curling up her knees toward her chest. "He thinks I'm your girl, doesn't he?" She giggled. "Isn't that funny?"

St. Louis had looked down into the baby's face; he supposed it *was* funny, imagining anybody as his girl. But he didn't feel like laughing. Instead, he was unable to prevent himself from leaning down and kissing the baby. The little lips puckered, but the eyelashes remained resolutely fastened to the baby's cheeks.

"You're sweet with him," Louise said after a minute, watching him from the bed. "What did you want him for so much, anyway?"

St. Louis watched the baby in his arms, the child's lips moving soundlessly. It looked as if he were speaking, repeating something over and over.

This was the hardest question, even harder than the one Louise had asked before, about how long he thought it would be before they caught up with him. He could make himself think about who might come, for there was a long list: Hoffman, and Alice—even the baby's aunt Evie, the aunt who'd shown up at the last minute.

Louise had been eager to report the particular details of the aunt's sudden arrival and explanations to St. Louis.

"You saw her," Louise had said to him that night when they sat on the terrace of the Café de la Paix. St. Louis had treated Louise to dinner, counting on her for information. "Wasn't she pretty? And she was educated, too; you could tell by the way she talked." Louise did an imitation. "'I'm here on behalf of my sister.' That's what she told Alice. And do you know what else?" Louise took a big mouthful of chocolate mousse—the café's specialty—and then reached across the table familiarly to wipe a crumb from St. Louis's cheek. "You'll never guess what happened to the father!"

"Oh, but I bet I would," St. Louis had said, and had surprised Louise by telling her about the young man with the hatbox.

"But what about the mother?" he'd asked Louise. "Where's the mother?"

Louise had wiped her mouth carefully. "I got the impression that the mother isn't completely sold on the idea of this baby. Not one hundred percent certain," she said. "Can you imagine? Can you imagine not being certain about your *own baby?*"

No, St. Louis had thought. He could not imagine it. And in

a way, that had decided it for him. All those orphans—he could have taken all those orphans. But someone *wasn't certain* about the hatbox baby.

How dare they, he'd thought. *How dare they.*

But Louise had said the aunt was determined—she'd take the baby if her sister was unwilling to raise him.

So even she might come, too, all the way to Pharaoh, Virginia, in search of her nephew.

And of course Caro herself would come now to find him out. A righteous anger flared up briefly in St. Louis at the thought of Caro, who had not helped him.

Or maybe they'd send the police.

The thought of policemen made him exhausted, an exhaustion he'd been putting away since leaving Chicago. The string of his crimes flew behind him, an evil black kite tail. It flew in the window and lay over the sill, flapping gently. St. Louis had to stop himself from slamming down the sash.

With a tremendous effort, he'd looked down at Louise and met her eyes. He found himself able to smile at her. Amazing: from where had he pulled that smile?

"My uncle Warren minds everything right now, I think," he heard himself say to Louise at last. "But it will be all right. Don't worry."

And at that, her question shivered and contracted like a leaf going up in flames. Another day. He'd think about it another day. Why had he stolen this baby? Why had he?

He'd hesitated at the door, the baby warm in his arms. "Thank you, Louise."

She waved at him with her eyes closed. "So long as I have my money, I wouldn't be mad," she said. "The fair was almost over, anyway." She yawned again. "Bring him back when he gets hungry. I don't mind waking up. God, I'm used to it."

On the hillside that night, as he lay at the periphery of the meadow out of reach of the slanting parallelogram of light that fell from the door over the tangled, overgrown lawn and broken-down apple tree, the little piece of flint that had stuck into him when Louise had asked him why he'd stolen the baby grew into a splinter. It fit itself under his skin and worried there.

On his chest, the baby sighed—a tiny breath—and then shuddered. St. Louis concentrated on the feel of the earth under his back, the weight of the baby over his heart. He put his lips to the baby's head, the throbbing pulse there.

"It's called the fontanel," Alice had told him, certain in her brisk white nurse's uniform, moving among the babies and the incubators like a whiskery old mammoth, her long teeth like tusks, her breath smelling unpleasantly of vegetables. Only a baby wouldn't notice how ugly Alice Vernon was.

St. Louis had liked doing magic for Alice. He wasn't good enough to do any in front of a real audience, but he loved to find someone who would sit still and let him make a few mistakes. Alice had been the perfect person—unused to attention from anyone, easily charmed by someone who didn't seem to notice how ugly she was, grateful. One night, as they'd stood together outside the baby house watching the storks, he had reached over and pulled a cone of paper flowers from behind her ear. She'd actually blushed.

Was it at that moment, that moment of extraordinary cruelty, that he knew he could do it? Could steal a baby right out from under Alice Vernon's ugly, watchful nose?

As ugly as he was, he could never have made love to anyone who was as ugly as Alice, as ugly as himself. It would have been laughable. The only women he'd ever had, he'd had to pay for, or they'd been so drunk they'd hardly noticed.

But now, at the thought of Alice standing miserable and enraged over the baby's empty bassinet, he felt what in some ways was the worst guilt he'd suffered yet. Taking the money had been nothing compared to this. Caro had too much money for her own good anyway; even she said so. No, this was worse, worse even than the grief he'd felt at leaving Caro at last, after all this time, for that was tempered with anger, too. And it was worse than the grief of finding Warren so ruined. But Alice— nothing could stitch up the hole in Alice.

St. Louis pressed his lips again to the baby's head, the fine hair there, and made an apology into the air, the thick layer of stars above him.

For three days now, he had held the baby close to his chest nearly every minute of the day and night, except when Louise had taken the baby to feed him. He was good at it; it didn't even seem an effort to him to hold the baby all the time. He never wanted to put him down at all. Alice had been proud of how St. Louis was with the babies, and even Hoffman, who made his rounds with a certain hauteur, had nodded at St. Louis's attentions to the babies. If Caro thought St. Louis was all right, Hoffman could make no objection to the man's coming and rocking the babies. The Coney Island hospital was full of rockers, as they called them, though all the rest were women, of course, not men; and St. Louis had heard Alice on the subject of how the babies needed to feel the touch of human hands, hear the sound of human voices.

St. Louis sighed. Still, he could not completely explain this final act, this theft of a human being, to anyone, even to himself. He hadn't even planned it exactly, not until the very end, when the baby's aunt had shown up.

Lying in the meadow grass now, St. Louis blinked up at the stars overhead, the buttery orb of the moon. A sharp, pungent scent wafted over them. Skunk, he recognized. He heard the deer cough once again; it was ranging even deeper into the woods, past the hexagonal bottling house, with its Oriental roof and glass windows, which Warren had built by the spring. Day's Lithia Water. Warren had made a good business from it once. What had happened to stop it up? Did springs do that? Just mysteriously dry up?

The miracle spring, St. Louis had called it. Warren had said it would cure you, and to St. Louis that had meant *of anything*. Of ugliness. Of being an orphan. But of course it couldn't.

The baby lying on his chest made a little noise—*ah! ah! ah!*—a small cry of apprehension, and St. Louis touched the child's cheek with his own rough finger, stroking the round curve. He'd helped Alice weigh the baby the night before he'd stolen it.

"Exactly five pounds and five ounces," Alice had said in satisfaction. "Well done, young man! Wait till we tell Dr. Hoffman! No one would ever try to put *you* in a hatbox now!"

But he had started in a hatbox, St. Louis knew. He had come to the fair in a hatbox, almost dead.

Somewhere nearby, a deer cracked through branches, and St. Louis felt under his back the distant report of its tiny hooves speeding away down the pasture. Above him, a fat cloud that was pushed against the moon now suddenly turned red. The baby's legs jerked spasmodically.

How could he be parted from his baby now?

A brace of new stars had appeared in the sky, a seam of diamonds running horizon to horizon. Far away in Chicago, the music swelled, the colored lights swung crazily over the lagoon, the jewel-collared leopard at the feet of the Ethiopian princess sprang up and paced against its tether, the crowds pressed together at the entrance to the fan dancer's show, and inside, Caro stepped into the blue smoke onstage behind her waving ostrich-feather fans.

St. Louis held the child close. How could he be parted from this baby?

Where in the whole wide world could he go now without his baby?

FIFTEEN

The light, St. Louis thought, looking up toward the hills the next morning, was the light of the kindest dream, gentle and hazy, steam from the blue meadows floating up into the clearing air. You could walk into it as into water, wading into the yellow grasses fringed with millions of droplets of dew already transforming into vapor, and be made finer by your immersion in the pure loveliness of daybreak over the mountains.

But the babies were crying, and Louise was banging pots in the kitchen, and Warren, thin and baffled and unsure, was pacing restlessly through the house, checking behind doors.

There was work to be done.

St. Louis had the tools for it. His own strong body, his two hands—clever and knowing with knots and saws, axes and scythes. And diapers, Louise reminded him. And diapers.

Together they swept and scrubbed and sponged down the walls. Warren, fed a breakfast of oatmeal and honey and made to bathe in buckets of icy water from the well, and then set to gathering apples fallen from the trees in front of the house in the sun, became placid and calm in a clean white collarless shirt. Louise shaved him with a blade St. Louis sharpened, and she trimmed his hair. She put her baby in his lap and set them to swing on the porch.

St. Louis cut the grass in front of the house, sending up clouds of tiny black grasshoppers that leaped away from his blade, making the grass whir and sing. Louise washed curtains, beat the rugs, fed the babies—one at each breast—lying in the hammock with an embroidered pillow under her head and a quilt over her legs.

Over the next three days, between tasks, St. Louis tied the hatbox baby to his chest in a sling made of an old sheet—to leave his hands free—and walked the farm in the heavy sunshine, becoming reacquainted with this place he had left so many years before. The swing hanging from the end of a fraying rope in the barn—he was amazed to find it so low to the ground. And the steps from the kitchen door—had he once been afraid to leap down them? There were only two, so low he could take them now in one stride.

One afternoon, surprising two tough, muscled brown hens running wild out behind the icehouse, he had knelt by the old stone foundation and peered underneath—had he once been small enough to crawl under there and find eggs?

He had. Once.

Everywhere he went he had the surprising sensation of feeling as though everything around him had grown mysteriously smaller. It made him feel he had grown larger. Everywhere he went, the baby held close to his heart, his hand folded protectively over the child's head, he had to stoop to pass under branches, or duck to avoid tools hung from the barn rafters, or stand perplexed—barred by his surprising new size—before secret, half-remembered, narrow paths between hedges.

Something had happened to change him. Once, he had been almost overlooked, the child who could fit himself into the narrow tunnels under the boxwoods, the boy familiar with the cellar under the barn or the floor beneath the bottling house. He remembered standing eye-level with the piano keyboard, watching his aunt's fingers depress the ivory keys. He remembered hiding under the bed, watching Caro's bare feet dancing over the floor at dusk. He remembered places of shadows and darkness, remembered finding the forgotten things of the household— thimbles that had rolled into crevices behind the sideboard, pencils that had fitted into the cracks of the floorboards, and once, an opal ring, fallen from his aunt's hand as she shelled peas, in the cool, moist earth under the back steps. The glinting white eye of the stone had stared up at him like the eye of the Cyclops, huge and unblinking.

Once, he had taken up no room at all. Once, he had been so small that the world had seemed beyond the compass of his imagining, a place without borders or limits, a place so huge that the sky, when he stood beneath it, had filled him with a mixture of dread and joy, the sense that he ought to bow before it, make obeisance to its vastness. That, at least, had not changed, he thought, standing beneath the stars at night, holding the hatbox baby in his arms. He felt as small then as he had ever felt. It was only when he forgot to look up, when he attended with a rare joy to everything on the farm that needed to be mended or repaired or polished or cut down, that he felt masterful. Here was eminence, he thought, lifting kettles of hot water for Louise to wash the bedding. Here was eminence, he thought, fitting in a new board across the porch.

Here—taking the hatbox baby in his arms—here was eminence.

But all the while he was counting the days. They would

come and take his baby. Even now, he thought, Caro and Hoffman could be disembarking from the train in Pharaoh, coughing up dust.

And then, when they have gone, he thought, *I will be only a shadow of what I had hoped to become, so small that I will have sped backward in time to when I was a child leaning over the spring and praying the impossible prayer that the miracle waters from the center of the earth would enter my body and make me whole.*

And yet he could not escape the pleasure he felt in what they accomplished every day. The fourth evening in Pharaoh, at five o'clock, just after supper, he and Louise sat at the scrubbed kitchen table, the babies lying in their dresser drawers on the floor beside them, and made a list of stores they would need. That afternoon, a stooped and balding neighbor, who explained that he looked in on Warren from time to time, had stopped by and stood on the porch, amazed at the transformation of the house and of Warren himself, who stepped forward cordially and shook the man's hand and introduced St. Louis.

"My nephew," he said, "come home."

The man had brought in sacks from the back of his truck— potatoes and flour, coffee and sugar, lamp oil, half a smoked ham, a pint of whiskey. Still, they would need so much more, St. Louis found himself thinking, tapping his pencil—nails and soap and butter and milk. Boards for the henhouse, and oil and gasoline for his uncle's truck. The roof over the porch needed mending. Two broken windows called for glass. He wanted potatoes to plant in the garden, and seed for winter crops. He wanted a rooster for the hens. He wanted . . . so many things.

"What's there to do around here at night?" Louise said finally, bored with list-making. "All this work during the day is fine, but can't we have even a little music at night?"

Warren, who had been idling at the door to the kitchen and watching their discussion with the expression of a man who has come home to find his barren house suddenly filled with elves, spoke up. "There's the radio."

St. Louis looked up at him.

"Works fine still," Warren said.

A few minutes later, he and Louise were in the parlor, turning the knobs—there was George Gershwin, playing his *Rhapsody in Blue*.

"Now, that's more like it," Louise said, delighted.

St. Louis left them and went back into the kitchen. The hat-box baby was not asleep but was lying quietly in his drawer, his eyes open. St. Louis bent down over him, touched a finger to his cheek. The baby turned his head instinctively at the touch. He did not yet focus on anything, though sometimes he stared up in the direction of St. Louis's face and gazed toward his eyes as if trying to find some entrance there.

St. Louis stooped and raised him in his arms.

"I'm going for a walk," he said into the parlor as he went past. Neither Louise nor Warren, intent on the radio, looked up after him, though Louise, when her own baby began to cry a minute or two later, stopped at the front door for a moment and saw St. Louis's figure, the baby in his arms, heading down through the glowing evening light of the meadow toward the edge of the woods.

"Now, where's he going?" she called back to Warren, who came to stand beside her at the door.

"That's where the spring used to be," Warren said, as they watched St. Louis leave the amber light and disappear into the darkness of the trees, onto a path marked with a stone post. "It's dried up. Went dry years ago." He pushed open the door. "It would cure what ailed you, though. We always told him that."

And then they both turned at the sound of an approaching car.

When Hoffman and Caro stood on the porch a few moments later, Louise was the only one left to meet them. Warren had vanished into the house, trembling. He would not speak to Caro.

It was as St. Louis had imagined a few nights before, when he lay hidden in the meadow. Words passed between Louise and Hoffman and Caro, though St. Louis was too far away to hear them, winding down the soft path through the woods toward the spring. Louise, weeping, did indeed raise her arm, as he had feared, and point down across the meadow. The sky had deepened now to a violent rose, the cooling air busy with an armada of swooping, sharp-winged bats and barn swallows traversing the waves of shadows, the grasses bristling with the last light.

St. Louis could not hear them as they turned and stepped down off the porch, as they crossed the gravel drive and entered the meadow, though if he had seen Caro coming first ahead of Hoffman, he would have remembered her queenlike procession through this same place so many years before, when she wore over her shoulders a sheet that trailed behind her in a long, virgin train, a wand of bright forsythia held high in her hand. Behind her had run a little boy, catching the grasshoppers that leaped away in her wake, his eyes at the ground she stepped over so lightly.

It was dark in the woods, a darkness filled with the smooth breathing noises of the wind in the trees and the hurrying away of birds and small animals. The ground beneath his feet twinkled with tiny stones and the soft, white, decaying wood of fallen branches, curls of birch bark, winking shade flowers —hooded yellow leaves, blue stars, silver buttons. Looking down, he thought of the fair as it had looked from the height of the Ferris wheel at night, a place of rich and astonishing detail, so beautiful and surprising and strange that you could not believe it was real, not until you had descended into its midst and seen the sun roll down the avenues and heard the music begin and you had taken the hand of chance outstretched toward your own and walked into the amazing present.

Somewhere in Chicago, he thought, as he held the child close and walked on, Madame Zenda was sitting on her barrel, warming the flame beneath her mystical potions, shaking out her crimson skirts, telling fortunes.

He thought of the hatbox baby's father—how long had he wandered around that day, blinded by the brilliance of the fair, so utterly in the dark?

Any minute now, he thought, he and the hatbox baby might find the spring, the stone font empty, still dried up. Or they might find it running with water again, restored.

It was never what you expected, your future.

All the way home from the fair on the afternoon she discovered that her nephew was still alive, was well and whole and wrapped in a white blanket, Evie had thought she would burst with her news. *I was right*, she said to herself as she fixed dinner that night and waited for Sylvie to come home. *He's alive. I was right.*

She unwrapped two pale pink pork chops from their brown paper wrapping, scrubbed potatoes and carrots, filled a pan with water and set it to boil, all the while thinking, *I was right, I was right.*

Buoyant with relief and imagining a celebration, she had splurged on dinner, her habitual financial caution swept away by the certainty of good fortune, a certainty that had presented itself simultaneously with the sight of the baby, so pink and perfect and tiny—and so like a baby, a real baby, not the imagined floating orphan of her dreams but someone specific now, a child with a future that would be intertwined with her own. With the fact of his survival, she and Sylvie—Aunt and Mother, they had become—had been ushered out from under the umbrella of tragedy and escorted into a bright ballroom the size and dimension of a stadium, where the lights blazed and music played, where people stepped up onto a threshold and were shown the amazing possibilities of happiness in all its forms, living postcards of prosperity and joy: glowing green lawns, and porch swings stirring, and front doors with polished knockers, and welcome mats that spoke when you put your heel on them and said *Enter. Take your place here, pick up your glass, and drink. You have not been forgotten.*

Working in the small kitchen of the apartment as the sun set that night, she was gracious with its shortcomings, for now it was only temporary. Her mind leaped ahead from the fact of the baby himself and raced on into a future furnished magically with every comfort. Here were her two old chipped plates, but soon she would wrap them up, put them away in a box, and one day, retrieving something from the attic of the house that would be theirs in the future—a gabled house, she thought, with bedrooms for them all, and a hat rack by the door, and a dog, yes, a little dog, brown with white spots, for the boy, for every boy must have a dog!—she would find them again and turn them in her hands and remember this moment, this day, when her prayers had been answered. Years of kneeling by her bed at night, and now, look, she had been heard.

I promise to be humble, she thought, suddenly afraid, pausing with the plates in her hands.

She assessed the plainness of the table and fetched her scarf from the bedroom for a tablecloth, replacing the plates on its flowered surface.

I promise not to forget this, she thought.

All around her, the smells of other people's dinners came in at the window—frying onions, and chicken carcasses boiling in pots, and browning beef marrow. She felt a stab of camaraderie with her neighbors, most of whom she did not know. She stood and looked out across the street. Behind every lighted window, people took their places at the table, despite this time of poverty and deprivation, despite the uncertainty and dread and fear, and broke bread together, a majestic act of thanksgiving.

But the evening wore on, and eventually, up and down the street, lights went out and her neighbors went to bed. Evie had a pork chop alone, sitting on the bed by the radio and eating with her fingers. She put the potatoes and the carrots and the other pork chop in a dish and set them aside. She turned out the light and sat on in the dark.

And still Sylvie did not come home.

Evie's joy flickered. Little shoes, she thought valiantly. His first haircut, his first prayer book—bone white and with a gold ribbon to mark his favorite psalms. His first suit. Christmas morning, and a train track around the tree. A bright-haired boy on a swing beneath an elm tree.

A boy who came too early and was lost and then found.

She sat on the bed and watched the street through the open window and summoned up the future, but it was slipping away from her, water in a sieve. The bedclothes beneath her were damp with her sweat, and the lights of the pictures she had held in her mind all afternoon and evening were fading. Over at the fairgrounds, Alice Vernon switched off the lamps in the baby house and patrolled the perimeter of the nursery, checking heartbeats. The storks in the garden of the incubator house ran wildly once at the fence, imagining escape.

At last Evie could not wait anymore. She stood up and left the apartment, carrying her happiness away with her like a match cupped against the wind. If she could find Sylvie before it went out altogether, before the day ended and the spell was broken—it was superstitious, she knew, but if she could not say it before the end of the day, it would be gone, the opportunity squandered, thrown away. She hurried away toward the movie house—where else could Sylvie be?—toward her sister in her high glass ticket box, which shone like a faraway stage suspended in the summer darkness. Under the bright lights, Sylvie's hair would be on fire, her face white as snow; untouchable behind her glass, she exuded a rare, mysterious beauty. In the movie house the black-and-white past ran on an eternal reel, everything approaching the end but then starting again so that you could have it all a second time, or a third, or a fourth, as many times as it took to get it right, as many times as you chose, riding the roller-coaster curve of hope and fear and relief over and over until it became your own life, and you whirled away within it, a captive.

And there she was.

From the sidewalk, where Evie stood in the shadow of a tree and hesitated in the warm, penetrating darkness of the street, she could see Sylvie in her illuminated glass ticket booth, a distant figure, a squat, bored idol on her makeshift throne, her round shoulders slumped, one hand held up before her mouth, which was opened in a yawn like a cat's, a pink hole laced with white teeth. Evie thought of the lighted pilothouses of the barges at night on Lake Michigan, their lonely captains afloat on the black water under the stars, beyond the reach of human voices, attending to the feel of the water below them, its pitch and wallow, its smell and sound, its depths and sudden, dangerous, grinding shallows.

The ruby-papered lobby behind Sylvie's glass booth was empty. Everyone was inside, watching the last few minutes of a story unfold, while Sylvie waited at the gate, not a heroine or a villain but only a ticket taker, hovering at the periphery of the world like a moth at the glass of a hurricane lamp.

Evie waited. The words rose and fell in her throat.

And then suddenly Sylvie stood up, a flutter of bills in her hand, a black metal cash box under one arm. She yawned again, and Evie saw her hitch her skirt, run her tongue over her teeth, pat her cheek briskly with her fingers. *Wake up*.

The bells in the church at the corner began to ring, the solemn hour of midnight. For a moment, as the clock struck, Sylvie hovered there in her booth, filling the lighted box that floated in the shadowy lobby; she was swelling to unimaginable proportions within it. Evie stepped out from under the branches of the tree into the light that fell over the sidewalk from the domed streetlamp, but she knew she stood there empty-handed. The present had already run on past her, a story whose course could not be interrupted now because it was already barreling away toward the future, doors opening and closing for the last time, flowers being thrown or suns setting or final looks being exchanged. All the horror and all the bright wonder and all the astonishing novelty of the ending was away, away down a long corridor of time.

And then Sylvie turned away in her glass booth, whose windows shone like ice, and a door opened at the back of the box, and she stepped down into the darkness and was gone.

Caro spoke first. "What's his name?"

Dr. Hoffman stopped in the tall grass of the meadow, leaned over, and took off his shoe, then shook it out and replaced it. "Whose?" he said. "Please, wait a minute."

She paused. "The baby's," she said finally. "What is the baby's *name*?"

Dr. Hoffman looked at her. "I don't know. He doesn't have one." He straightened up and stood there, bewildered, his shoe-lace dangling. All this talk. All this back and forth. All this struggling over how they should proceed, what was right, let alone what authority he might have to decide the baby's fate finally, and *the baby had no name*. The questions of the last few days buzzed inside his head. The child's aunt had not returned to the nursery since St. Louis and Louise had run off, so she did not know of the theft, presumably, but Alice felt sure she would come back. And what would she want then? If the mother herself did not want the child, was not the aunt entitled? Did the aunt want the baby for herself? Surely a court of law would say blood was the defining issue here. And what about punishment?

What about another baby, Caro had asked him. If not this one, what about one of the ones no one wanted?

But there had been a theft, he reminded himself, thinking slowly, a theft of a human child.

And yet, why was it his own shame he felt now?

All this, and the baby had no name. Or none that they knew.

How tentative everything was, Dr. Hoffman thought. How provisional and unclear, everything held in a kind of abeyance. There was some method of discovery here, he sensed, some shaping of events that would carry them all into the future, but right now he did not know how to proceed.

"Wait," Caro had said to him on the train. "Please, Leo. Talk to him. Just wait until we get there."

"We never named him," he said now, staring at Caro. "No one ever named him."

They stood together, and after a while they looked away from each other and into the blackening line of trees before them.

On the train, as they had sat across from each other hour after hour, holding hands over their knees, Caro had argued for time.

"Who are we," she had said to him, "to decide how it should end?"

And he'd had no answer for her.

At last he reached over and tugged her to sit down beside him. The sun fell away behind High Peak. Louise came out of the house and stood on the porch, a lantern in one hand, her baby held against her shoulder, watching Dr. Hoffman and Caro as they sat side by side in the tall grass.

Fireflies rose in a swarm over their heads. Stars filled the sky. The moon lifted free of the trees, filling the meadow with the pale light of benediction. Even as they watched, the sky seemed to change over their heads, the stars forming themselves into new shapes.

"What are we doing?" Caro said at last.

"Shhh," Dr. Hoffman said, and he heard the wind pick up and come toward them on little feet. "Listen. We're waiting."

AUTHOR'S NOTE
AND ACKNOWLEDGMENTS

◼

The public exhibition at fairs and expositions of live premature babies in incubators was common around the turn of the century, both in the United States and in Europe. One physician engaged in such practices, perhaps the most notable among them, was Dr. Martin A. Couney. Born in Alsace in 1860 or 1870 (accounts differ), he was educated in Breslau, Berlin, Leipzig, and Paris, where he studied with Professor Pierre Constant Budin, a leading pediatrician who helped pioneer efforts to save prematurely born infants. Couney's obituary in the *New York Times* reports his death in March of 1950.

In addition to his work at world's fairs, Dr. Couney was also known for his Infantorium, as it was called, on Coney Island, where he charged admission to his hospital for the prematurely born (and where Archibald Leach, who went on to metamorphose into the famous Cary Grant, reportedly was a barker, patrolling the boardwalk and encouraging passersby to stop in and see the babies). Dr. Couney used the proceeds from public admissions to run his hospital and advance his considerable medical research. Few hospitals were offering expert care for premature infants at the time; many, especially in New York, referred infants to Couney.

Dr. Couney never charged parents for his medical attentions to their babies, though his care was often prolonged, sometimes lasting several months until the infants were strong enough to go home to their families.

"I made propaganda for the preemies," Dr. Couney is said to have concluded at the time of his retirement, and we are meant to take the word *propaganda* in the best way possible.

Today, however, the notion of such exhibits strikes us as the height of bad taste, at the least, and as inhumane, at the worst. Yet it appears that Dr. Couney's motives were good, his medical practices sound, and his methods of public education effective, though unconventional by today's standards. A. J. Liebling, who wrote about Dr. Couney for the *New Yorker* in 1939, established that the doctor was widely admired by his peers in the medical establishment, who credited him with saving the lives of thousands of children who arrived too early in the world and might otherwise have died without Dr. Couney's knowledgeable intervention.

I am indebted to the work of William A. Silverman, M.D., who researched Dr. Couney's life and practices and published (among other works) a long article on Couney in the journal *Pediatrics* in 1979, for a description of Dr. Couney's life and work, as well as speculations about the doctor's motives and character.

My own creation for the purposes of this novel, Dr. Leo Hoffman, borrows many biographical details from Dr. Couney's life but is in no way intended as a reflection of Dr. Couney's character, about which I, like Dr. Silverman, can offer only sympathetic speculation. This novel is not, in that sense, strictly a historical novel but is more generally inspired by history and the figures who populated the past. Dr. Leo Hoffman is not intended to be read as a portrait of Dr. Couney, per se, but as the study of a man involved with the same dynamic and complex circumstances that surrounded Dr. Couney himself. To maintain a respectful distance between Dr. Couney and the man I imagined, I chose to rename the character and to alter freely some material facts of Dr. Couney's life in creating Dr. Hoffman's. Dr. Hoffman is, for instance, considerably younger than Dr. Couney himself would have been at the 1933 fair in Chicago.

Real people, their characters and characteristics, are always the basis of fiction's interest in human affairs. To Dr. Couney, whose life and work inspired me and gave me entrance into the novel, I offer the tribute of my enduring fascination.

Dr. Couney did have an exhibit at the 1933 Century of Progress Exposition in Chicago, as well as at Earl's Court in London in the late nineteenth century and at various other fairs in the United States up to and into the 1940s. I have used details from the 1933 Chicago exhibition as well as others to create the one imagined for this novel. It is true that Dr. Couney's Chicago exhibition was located near the famous fan dancer Sally Rand, but the fictional character of Caroline Day, who is the fan dancer in the novel, bears no relation, or only accidental relation, to Sally Rand herself, about whom I know next to nothing.

Dr. Couney had an important colleague in Chicago, Dr. Julius H. Hess, who became a respected expert on premature babies. For the novel's purposes, I invented the fictional Dr. Elliott Ludwig, but he owes only his time and place to Hess, and nothing to his character, about which I know as much as I do about Sally Rand.

The character of St. Louis Percy is entirely a fictional invention, as are the other characters in the story. Notably, A. J.

Liebling reports an anecdote about a man approaching Dr. Couney with a hatbox that contained a live baby at the Omaha Trans-Mississippi Exposition in 1898, but there is no evidence that such deliveries were common or that one occurred at Chicago's Century of Progress.

Though it is a fairly simple matter to demarcate the line between fact and fiction in regard to the characters of the novel, the extent to which the fair I imagined is a true reflection of the actual Century of Progress is a more complex matter. The writer Thomas Mallon has used this phrase to accommodate the necessary liberties he takes with truth to invent a purposeful fictional universe: "Nouns always trump adjectives, and in the phrase 'historical fiction' it is important to remember which of the two words is which." I am indebted to Mallon for this axiom, and for his example of willful and inspired distortion.

I am also indebted to the Chicago Historical Society for the use of its archival records of the 1933 Century of Progress Exposition and to the many journalists of the time who wrote about the fair for diverse venues.

I read widely in the pages of the *Chicago Tribune* for the summer months of 1933 for a sense of the city at that time and its role as civic host to the fair. The fair itself and its original board of directors generated many invaluable documents, maps, drawings, and photographs, which have helped me to imagine a place and time that no longer exists. I have also from time to time deliberately borrowed from accounts of other fairs or invented from my own imagination details that seemed helpful in establishing verisimilitude. Despite these deviations from the "truth," I have tried to present an overall impression of the fair—strange and wondrous and perplexing as it was—in as accurate a light as possible.

I would like to thank both Lisa Johnston and Joe Malloy of the Sweet Briar College Library, who showed themselves to be tireless and resourceful pursuers of information. For their enthusiasm and assistance while I was researching this novel, I am deeply grateful.

My thanks also to Dr. Allen Majewski and the nursing staff at the Neonatal Intensive Care Unit of Virginia Baptist Hospital in Lynchburg, Virginia, for answering my many questions.

To Dr. William Brown, for telling me about the four elements, for careful reading of the manuscript, and for his own intuitive and sympathetic brand of medicine, I am especially thankful.

I would also like to thank the Virginia Commission for the Arts for a grant that helped support me while I worked on this book.

CARRIE BROWN